This book is due for return on or before the last date shown below

2 3 APR 2014
- 1 SEP 2016

O A R L
OXFORD AMERICAN RHEUMATOLOGY LIBRARY

Rheumatoid Arthritis

Michael H. Weisman, MD

Director, Division of Rheumatology
Professor of Medicine
Cedar-Sinai Medical Center
Professor Emeritus of Medicine
University of California (UCSD) School of Medicine
San Diego, CA

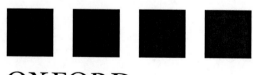

OXFORD
UNIVERSITY PRESS
2011

OXFORD
UNIVERSITY PRESS

Oxford University Press, Inc., publishes works that further
Oxford University's objective of excellence
in research, scholarship, and education.

Oxford New York

Auckland Cape Town Dar es Salaam Hong Kong Karachi
Kuala Lumpur Madrid Melbourne Mexico City Nairobi
New Delhi Shanghai Taipei Toronto

With offices in
Argentina Austria Brazil Chile Czech Republic France Greece
Guatemala Hungary Italy Japan Poland Portugal Singapore
South Korea Switzerland Thailand Turkey Ukraine Vietnam

Copyright © 2011 by Oxford University Press, Inc.

Published by Oxford University Press, Inc.
198 Madison Avenue, New York, New York 10016

www.oup.com

Oxford is a registered trademark of Oxford University Press

Library of Congress Cataloging-in-Publication Data

Weisman, Michael H.
Rheumatoid arthritis / Michael H. Weisman.
p. ; cm. — (Oxford American rheumatology library)
Includes bibliographical references and index.
ISBN 978-0-19-975421-2 (standard ed. : alk. paper)
1. Rheumatoid arthritis—Diagnosis. 2. Rheumatoid arthritis—Treatment.
I. Title. II. Series: Oxford American rheumatology library.
[DNLM: 1. Arthritis, Rheumatoid—diagnosis. 2. Arthritis, Rheumatoid—drug therapy.
3. Diagnosis, Differential. 4. Outcome Assessment (Health Care) WE 346 W428r 2011]
RC933.W435 2011
616.7'227—dc22   2010013597

Disclosures

Dr. Weisman has nothing to disclose.

Contents

Chapter 1

History of Rheumatoid Arthritis

The origins and early history of rheumatoid arthritis (RA) are difficult to ascertain and subject to both speculation and empirical analysis. There are those that argue that RA is a disease of the New World that was transmitted to the Old World by European explorers and settlers,[1] whereas others argue that RA was not unique to the New World and existed in the Old World in pre-Columbian populations.[2] Rothschild notes that RA "was first detected in the west branch of the Tennessee and Green Rivers, remained geographically localized for 5,000 years, and disseminated into Ohio 1,000 years ago".[3]

The results of two paleopathological studies appear to support the conclusion that RA is a disease of the New World. First, an analysis of the data from New World and Old World skeletal remains, some dating as far back as 6,500 years, revealed that only the skeletal remains of pre-Columbian North Americans met the accepted criteria for RA, with spondyloarthropathy being the most likely diagnosis for the majority of the Old World skeletal remains.[3] Second, an analysis of the skeletal remains of 613 individuals in Italy dating from the 16th century BCE to the 15th century CE concluded that there is no evidence that RA's existence in skeletal remains would be unmistakable—therefore it is unlikely the disease existed in the Old World at or before this time.[4]

Dequeker cites several examples of paintings by artists of the Flemish school, completed during the mid 15th to early 16th centuries, that hint at the presence of rheumatoid-like lesions in the European models used by these artists.[5] Although Dequeker's thesis is thought-provoking, it remains controversial because the deformities depicted in these paintings may be just as easily attributable to other conditions or to idealized conventions of particular schools of art.[6]

Although the first discussion of RA in contemporary medical literature is attributed to A.J. Landré-Beauvais, an earlier reference is the 1676 publication by Thomas Sydenham titled *Medical Observations Concerning the History and the Cure of Acute Diseases*, in which Sydenham quite accurately described the signs and symptoms of RA.[7] In his doctoral dissertation, published in 1800, A.J. Landré-Beauvais identified primary asthenic gout and proposed that primary asthenic gout should be distinguished from generalized gout, a generic term heretofore used to refer to specific diseases of the joints and rheumatism.[8] Although Landré-Beauvais was responsible for the initial work leading to the disentanglement of RA from other forms of joint disease, it wasn't until the late 1800s that the term *rheumatoid arthritis* was introduced. Sir Alfred Baring Garrod proposed the term to designate "an inflammatory affectation of the joints, not unlike rheumatism in some of its characters, but differing materially in its pathology".[9] Ultimately, in 1907, Sir Alfred Barring's son, Sir Archibald, made the distinction between osteoarthritis and RA.[10] The official designation of RA was adopted by the British Ministry of Health in 1922 and by the American Rheumatism Association (now the American College of Rheumatology) in 1941.

Within the last several decades, a wealth of new research findings have been reported that illuminate our understanding of the specific biological and molecular characteristics of RA. Commonalities among RA patients include the presence of rheumatoid factors and the occurrence of the disease among family members. The identification of rheumatoid factors led to the classification of RA as an autoimmune disease, while the search for a genetic basis for RA uncovered the HLA-DRB1 polymorphism that predicts onset, severity, and disease pattern. Antibodies, such as the anticitrullinated protein, are at the core of current thinking about the pathogenesis of RA, and have been discovered in the blood of RA patients well before disease onset.[11] The identification of rheumatoid factors, antibodies, and allelic polymorphisms is the foundation for the current research agenda in RA, which focuses on exploring gene–environment interactions and refining our understanding of the pathogenesis of RA.

Table 1.1 Milestones in the History and Identification of Rheumatoid Arthritis (RA)

Year/Milestone	Finding
Pre-Columbian Old World (Europe)	Analysis of skeletal remains not consistent with criteria for establishing the presence of RA. Disease most likely spondyloarthropathy.
Pre-Columbian North America	Analysis of skeletal remains consistent with current criteria for establishing the presence of RA.
15th to 17th century	Hands of models by painters of the Flemish school suggest presence of RA-type lesions.
1800	Dissertation of AJ Landré-Beauvais separates RA from gout as a unique disease.
1875	Sir Alfred Baring proposes the term *rheumatoid arthritis*.
1907	Sir Archibald Baring distinguishes osteoarthritis from RA.
1922	British Ministry of Health officially adopts the designation of RA.
1940 onward	Science of immunology introduced to the study of RA. Discovery of rheumatoid factors.
1941	American Rheumatism Association (now the American College of Rheumatology) officially adopts the designation of RA.
1960–1970 onward	Reports of highly specific antibodies for RA appear. Research focuses on anti-citrullinated peptide antibodies (ACPAs).
Early 1970s	Rheumatoid arthritis and rheumatoid spondylitis, previously thought to be an arthritis of the spine, distinguished as separate diseases. RA antibodies were not present in patients with spondylitis.
Late 1970s onward	Possible role of genetic factors explored. HLA-DRB1 associated with disease onset and severity.
2000 and beyond	Research focused on gene–environment interactions.

References

1. Buchanan WW. Rheumatoid arthritis: Another New World disease? *Semin Arthritis Rheum* 1994;23(5): 289–294.

2. Leden I, Arcini C. Doubts about rheumatoid arthritis as a New World disease. *Semin Arthritis Rheum* 1994;23(5):354–365.

3. Rothschild BM. Rheumatoid arthritis at a time of passage. *J Rheumatol* 2001;28(2): 245–250.

4. Rothschild BM, Coppa A, Petrone PP. "Like a virgin": Absence of rheumatoid arthritis and treponematosis, good sanitation and only rare gout in Italy prior to the 15th century. *Reumatismo* 2004; 56(1):61–66.

5. Dequeker J. Arthritis in Flemish paintings (1400–1700). *Br Med J.* 1977;1(6070):1203–1205.

6. Kahn M. The antiquity of rheumatoid arthritis. *Ann Rheum Dis.* 1993;52(4):316.

7. Short CL. The antiquity of rheumatoid arthritis. *Arthritis Rheum* 1974;17(3):193–205.

8. Landré-Beauvais AJ. The first description of rheumatoid arthritis. Unabridged text of the doctoral dissertation presented in 1800. *Joint Bone Spine* 2001;68(2):130–143.

9. Garrod AB. A treatise on gout and rheumatic gout. In *Rheumatoid Arthritis*, 3rd ed. London: Longmans, Green, 1875.

10. Symmons, DPM. What is rheumatoid arthritis? *Br. Med Bull* 1995;51(2):243–248.

11. Rantapaa-Dahlqvist S, de Jong BA, Berglin E, et al. Antibodies against cyclic citrullinated peptide and IgA rheumatoid factor predict the development of rheumatoid arthritis. *Arthritis Rheum* 2003;48(10):2741–2749.

Chapter 2

Definition and Classification

Definition

The National Cancer Institute accurately describes rheumatoid arthritis (RA) as "an autoimmune disease that causes pain, swelling, and stiffness in the joints, and may cause severe joint damage, loss of function, and disability. The disease may last from months to a lifetime, and symptoms may improve and worsen over time".[1] RA can appear in the upper extremities, lower extremities, and spine and axial joints, with characteristics including:[2]

- Inflammation (joint swelling with characteristic soft tissue involvement)
- Polyarthritis (involvement of >5 joints)
- Symmetry (same joint regions of both upper and lower extremities)
- Chronicity (duration of >6 weeks)
- Autoantibodies (RF, anti-CCP, anti-RA33)
- Erosions (bony destruction seen on conventional x-ray)
- Absence of recent infections or comorbid conditions associated with arthritides
- Painful metacarpophalangeal (MCP) or metatarsophalangeal (MTP) compression
- Morning stiffness (lasting more than a few minutes)
- Genetics

The disease process may be characterized as having four distinct phases: an initial phase in which there is no clinical evidence of the disease but some patients may have markers in the blood that denote autoimmunity; an early inflammatory phase that includes clinical manifestations that may or may not be accompanied by a confirmed diagnosis of RA; a destructive phase that includes erosions and disease progression; and an ongoing phase accompanied by irreversible joint destruction.[3] Simultaneously, there are two overlapping subpopulations of patients with RA: individuals who are positive for the presence of rheumatoid factor (RF), and individuals who are positive for the presence of antibodies that can bind cyclic citrullinated peptides (CCP).[4] Patients with either of these biomarkers tend to have a more severe course of RA, with anti-CCP antibodies having a greater prognostic value than RF.[4] Patients with neither of these biomarkers tend to have a more benign course and are referred to as having "seronegative" RA.

Rheumatoid arthritis progression and the pace of joint destruction are quite variable. SE+ DR4 alleles, RF production, gender, and the presence of erosive disease at presentation are among the factors that may influence the pace of joint destruction in RA, independent of inflammatory disease activity.[5]

Disease Onset

In an ideal world, the clinician would have a set of clinical, serological, and genetic markers at his or her disposal to determine which patients presenting with undifferentiated arthritis will go on to develop confirmed cases of RA. Unfortunately, at present, no clinical, serological, and genetic markers can predict which patients will develop RA. One avenue of current rheumatology research is devoted to the identification of RA prior to symptom onset. Several studies of the mechanisms of the RA pre-disease process have documented the presence of autoantibodies and the inflammatory marker C-reactive protein (CRP) in the bloodstream several years prior to a confirmed diagnosis of RA.[6–10] Although promising, this research is still in its infancy, and clinicians cannot rely on a model of pre-disease processes to identify patients likely to develop RA.

The clinician faced with a patient who presents with an undifferentiated arthritis or early synovitis is challenged to accurately diagnose and treat that patient before irreversible changes (damage) or a significant functional disability develop. The challenge is to distinguish these patients from those whose signs and symptoms of early synovitis will spontaneously remit. Under the direction of the American College of Rheumatology (ACR) and the European League Against Rheumatism (EULAR), major efforts are under way to identify patients with early inflammatory arthritis amenable to treatment, so that the disease does not progress to meet currently established ACR classification criteria (discussed below). By the time a patient meets ACR classification criteria, it is felt to be "too late" in the clinical evolution of the disease. The ACR/EULAR criteria, designed to distinguish patients with a high probability of having RA from those whose condition will likely remit and not need aggressive management, include which joints (and how many of them) are involved, serologic studies, duration of signs and symptoms, and acute phase proteins.[11] At present, there are no definitive cut-points as the process is still evolving. However, it is important to point out that there are many patients with persistent and disabling arthritis that does not fulfill the ACR classification criteria; these patients should be treated, and the new criteria will go a long way toward helping clinicians with this important decision.

In a patient with recent-onset synovitis or arthritis, it is also important to make certain that the synovitis or arthritis is not a primary infection—fungal, Lyme, or tuberculosis—and that the patient receives a workup for viral infections such as rubella, parvovirus, hepatitis, or HIV. Nevertheless, there is a need to identify patients with this early synovitis who will or have the potential to develop a destructive polyarthritis. Our primary goal should be to prevent these complications and treat these patients as soon as possible, while avoiding unnecessary interventions in patients with another disease or whose symptoms will spontaneously remit.[12] In some cases, a cut-off of greater than

6 weeks of disease duration will designate those patients who are destined to have established RA.[13]

Classification

It is imperative to diagnose and initiate treatment for RA as soon as possible in order to impede the disease process and hinder progression to major damage. The most widely used and recognized classification criteria for rheumatoid arthritis are the 1987 RA classification criteria of the American College of Rheumatology. These criteria were developed based on established disease and have a sensitivity of 91% and a specificity of 89%.[14] It is important to note that these criteria should be used for classification purposes only for patients with confirmed RA.

Classification criteria must straddle the balance between the requirement for specificity in clinical trial designs and the sensitivity required by physicians making clinical judgments. Classification criteria are typically very specific and provide methodological standardization for clinical study designs. As a result, sensitivity is sacrificed. For example, genetic studies of disease susceptibility require the specificity inherent in classification criteria to avoid misclassification. On the other hand, diagnosing patients requires sensitivity to a reasonable probability of disease presence in order to identify and "not miss" as many true positives as possible. In this case, specificity is sacrificed in favor of making the "right" diagnosis, leading to the identification of patients who may not have the disease (i.e., false positives). Until patients can be identified as definitely fulfilling the 1987 RA classification criteria, most rheumatologists feel that those not meeting the criteria should be identified as having "early synovitis," since a variable percentage of these "early" patients may have self-limited disease or evolve into another disease category. The 1987 RA classification criteria of the American College of Rheumatology[15] are provided in Table 2.1. The new proposed criteria[11] are an attempt to avoid the stringency of the 1987 criteria and permit classification decisions to be made at an earlier stage of the disease.

Table 2.1 1987 Criteria for the Classification of Acute Arthritis of Rheumatoid Arthritis

1. Morning stiffness	Morning stiffness in and around the joints, lasting at least 1 hour before maximal improvement
2. Arthritis of three or more joint areas	At least three joint areas simultaneously have had soft tissue swelling or fluid (not bony overgrowth alone) observed by a physician. The 14 possible areas are right or left PIP, MCP, wrist, elbow, knee, ankle, and MTP joints
3. Arthritis of hand joints	At least one area swollen (as defined above) in a wrist, MCP, or PIP joint
4. Symmetric arthritis	Simultaneous involvement of the same joint areas (as defined in 2) on both sides of the body (bilateral involvement of PIPs, MCPs, or MTPs is acceptable without absolute symmetry)

(continued)

Table 2.1 Continued	
5. Rheumatoid nodules	Subcutaneous nodules, over bony prominences, or extensor surfaces, or in juxtaarticular regions, observed by a physician
6. Serum rheumatoid factor	Demonstration of abnormal amounts of serum rheumatoid factor by any method for which the result has been positive in <5% of normal control subjects
7. Radiographic changes	Radiographic changes typical of RA on posteroanterior hand and wrist radiographs, which must include erosions or unequivocal bony decalcification localized in or most marked adjacent to the involved joints (osteoarthritis changes alone do not qualify)

For classification purposes, a patient shall be said to have rheumatoid arthritis if he/she has satisfied at least four of these seven criteria. Criteria 1 through 4 must have been present for at least 6 weeks. Patients with two clinical diagnoses are not excluded. Designation as classic, definite, or probable rheumatoid arthritis is *not* to be made.

PIP, proximal interphalangeal joint; **MCP**, metacarpophalangeal joint; **MTP**, metatarsophalangeal joint

References

1. http://www.cancer.gov/Templates/db_alpha.aspx?CdrID=455398.

2. Machold KP, Smolen JS. Early (rheumatoid) arthritis. In: Hochberg MC, et al., eds., *Rheumatoid Arthritis*, 1st edition. Philadelphia: Mosby 2009:73–81.

3. VanderBorght A, Geusens P, Raus J, Stinissen P. The autoimmune pathogenesis of rheumatoid arthritis: Role of autoreactive T cells and new immunotherapies. *Semin Arthritis Rheum* 2001;31(3):160–175.

4. Klareskog L, Padyukov L, Lorentzen J, Alfredsson L. Mechanisms of disease: Genetic susceptibility and environmental triggers in the development of rheumatoid arthritis. *Nat Clin Pract Rheumatol* 2006;2(8):425–433.

5. Kaltenhäuser S, Wagner U, Schuster E, et al. Immunogenetic markers and seropositivity predict radiological progression in early rheumatoid arthritis independent of disease activity. *J Rheumatol* 2001;28(4):735–744.

6. Aho K, Heliovaara M, Maatela J, et al. Rheumatoid factors antedating clinical rheumatoid arthritis. *J Rheumatol* 1991;18(9):1282–1284.

7. Aho K, von Essen R, Kurki P, et al. Antikeratin antibody and antiperinuclear factor as markers for subclinical rheumatoid disease process. *J Rheumatol* 1993;20(8):1278–1281.

8. Nielen MM, van Schaardenburg D, Reesink HW, et al. Specific autoantibodies precede the symptoms of rheumatoid arthritis: A study of serial measurements in blood donors. *Arthritis Rheum* 2004;50(2):380–386.

9. Rantapaa-Dahlqvist S, de Jong BA, Berglin E, et al. Antibodies against cyclic citrullinated peptide and IgA rheumatoid factor predict the development of rheumatoid arthritis. *Arthritis Rheum* 2003;48(10):2741–2749.

10. Symmons DPM. What is rheumatoid arthritis? *Br. Med Bull* 1995;51(2):243–248.

11. Aletaha D, Neogi T, Silman AJ, et al. The 2010 Classification Criteria for Rheumatoid Arthritis: an ACR/EULAR Collaborative Initiative. *Arthritis Rheum/ Ann Rheum Dis* 2010. In press.

12. Symmons D, Hazes, J, Silman AJ. Cases of early inflammatory polyarthritis should not be classified as having rheumatoid arthritis. *J Rheumatol* 2003;30(5):902–904.

13. Nielen MM, van Schaardenburg D, Reesink HW, et al. Increased levels of C-reactive protein in serum from blood donors before the onset of rheumatoid arthritis. *Arthritis Rheum* 2004;50(8):2423–2427.

14. Aletaha D, Breedveld FC, Smolen JS. The need for new classification criteria for rheumatoid arthritis. *Arthritis Rheum* 2005 Nov;52(11):3333–3336.

15. Arnett FC, Edworthy SM, Bloch DA, et al. The American Rheumatism Association 1987 revised criteria for the classification of rheumatoid arthritis. *Arthritis Rheum* 1988;31(3):315–324.

Chapter 3

Epidemiology

The presence of rheumatoid arthritis (RA) in any given population is measured by incidence and prevalence, where incidence is the number of new cases reported during a specified time period and prevalence is the number of current cases at any given time. The number of people affected by RA is relatively small. In the United States, the *prevalence* of RA has been declining over the last several decades, and is now estimated to be 0.6% of the population aged ≥18 years.[1] In European countries, the prevalence of RA has been reported to be as low as <0.2% in Yugoslavia[2] and as high as 0.8% in the United Kingdom.[3]

The *incidence* of RA across the world is also variable. The lowest rates have been reported in Japan and France, where the incidence rates are 8 per 100,000[4] and 8.8 per 100,000,[5] respectively. The highest incidence rate is in the United States, where the average annual age- and sex-adjusted incidence of RA is 44.6 per 100,000.[6] Rheumatoid arthritis incidence rates may fluctuate slightly, as they are affected by time of reporting and the gap between symptom onset and notification to a population-based registry.[7]

Ethnicity

The prevalence of RA is higher among Mexican Americans compared to both blacks and whites,[8] and the prevalence of RA among blacks is lower compared to whites.[9] Although the prevalence of RA among the black population is lower, there is no evidence that the disease expression itself differs,[9] and there is even some evidence to suggest that RA in blacks is less severe in terms of disability and presence of extra-articular manifestations.[10]

Several American Indian tribes and Alaska Native populations experience a much higher RA prevalence rate than their Caucasian counterparts. The prevalence rate of RA among the Chippewa Indians, for example, ranges from 6.8% to 7.1%, and the prevalence rate for Pima Indians is 5.3%. The Tlingit Indians also have a notably high prevalence rate (2.4%), and both Tlingit women and Yakima Indian women have similarly high prevalence rates, 3.5% and 3.4%, respectively.[11]

Sex

Rheumatoid arthritis is more common in women and uncommon in young men (<35 years). Data from the Rochester, Minnesota, incidence study in the United States show that there were a total of 609 incident cases, including 445 women and 164 men in an inception cohort first diagnosed between January 1, 1955 and

December 31, 1994, and followed-up until January 1, 2000. The incidence rate for women and men was 57.8 per 100,000 and 30.4 per 100,000, respectively.[6]

Data from the Third National Health and Nutrition Examination Survey (NHANES III) in the Unites States indicate that the prevalence of RA in women ranged from 2.35 to 2.71 per 100, whereas the prevalence of RA in men ranged from 1.59 to 1.85 per 100.[8]

A study of a prospective cohort of women in the Nurses' Health Study in the United States found significant regional variation in incident cases of RA even after controlling for confounding factors.[12] For example, RA risk was higher in women living in the eastern United States compared with women living in the western United States at birth, age 15 years, and age 30 years.

Age

For both men and women, the incidence of RA increases with age, although the peak incidence for women occurs earlier than the peak incidence for men. Prevalence also increases with age, as new cases in younger people are added to the "prevalence pool".[13] The NHANES III investigators used three different case identification strategies to estimate RA prevalence among people ≥60.[8] These case identification strategies yielded an RA prevalence between 2.03 per 100 and 2.34 per 100 among those aged 60 and older. Among those 60–69 years, prevalence ranged from 1.59 to 1.89 per 100 and, for those aged 70 and older, RA prevalence ranged from 2.46 to 2.8 per 100.

Trends

There is some evidence that the incidence of RA in the United States is declining. For example, the most recent data from the Rochester, Minnesota, study indicates that between 1955 and 1995, the incidence of RA declined from 61.2/100,000 person-years to 32.7/100,000-person years, with the decline significantly higher in women.[6]

Mortality

Although RA is not a fatal disease, data shows a gap in mortality between individuals with RA and the general population. Gonzalez et al. found that, although there have been improvements in the overall rate of mortality in the general U.S. population, RA patients have not been the beneficiaries of similar improvement.[14] This mortality gap seems to be confined to rheumatoid factor (RF) positive RA patients and is attributable primarily to cardiovascular and respiratory deaths.[15] There is growing attention being paid to an increased burden of cardiovascular disease in RA leading to the suggestion that more effective cardiovascular prevention and management is needed in RA treatment algorithms.[16]

References

1. Helmick CG, Felson DT, Lawrence RC, et al. Estimates of the prevalence of arthritis and other rheumatic conditions in the United States. *Arthritis Rheum* 2008;58(1):15–25.

2. Stojanovic R, Vlajinac H, Palic-Obradovic D, et al. Prevalence of rheumatoid arthritis in Belgrade, Yugoslavia. *Br J Rheumatol* 1998; 37(7):729–732.

3. Symmons D, Turner G, Webb R, et al. The prevalence of rheumatoid arthritis in the United Kingdom: New estimates for a new century. *Rheumatology* 2002;41(7):793–800.

4. Shichikawa K, Inoue K, Hirota S, et al. Changes in the incidence and prevalence of rheumatoid arthritis in Kamitonda, Wakayama, Japan, 1965–1996. *Ann Rheum Dis* 1999;58(12):751–756.

5. Guillemin F, Briancon S, Klein JM, et al. Low incidence of rheumatoid arthritis in France. *Scan J Rheumatol* 1994;23(5):264–268.

6. Doran MF, Pond GR, Crowson CS, et al. Trends in incidence and mortality in rheumatoid arthritis in Rochester, Minnesota, over a forty-year period. *Arthritis Rheum* 2002;46(3):625–631.

7. Wiles N, Symmons DP, Harrison B, et al. Estimating the incidence of rheumatoid arthritis: Trying to hit a moving target? *Arthritis Rheum* 1999;42(7):1339–1346.

8. Rasch EK, Hirsch R, Paulose-Ram R, Hochberg MC. Prevalence of rheumatoid arthritis in persons 60 years of age and older in the United States: Effect of different methods of case classification. *Arthritis Rheum* 2003;48(4):917–926.

9. Mikuls TR, Kazi S, Cipher D, et al. The association of race and ethnicity with disease expression in male US veterans with rheumatoid arthritis. *J Rheumatol* 2007;34(7):1480–1484.

10. Anaya JM, Rosler D, Espinoza LR. Rheumatoid arthritis in black Americans. *Ann Rheum Dis* 1994;53(11):782–783.

11. Ferucci ED, Templin DW, Lanier AP. Rheumatoid arthritis in American Indians and Alaska Natives: A review of the literature. *Semin Arthritis Rheum* 2005;34(4):662–667.

12. Costenbader KH, Chang SC, Laden F, et al. Geographic variation in rheumatoid arthritis incidence among women in the United States. *Arch Intern Med* 2008;168(15):1664–1670.

13. Silman AJ, Hochberg MC. Descriptive epidemiology of rheumatoid arthritis. In Hochberg MC, et al., eds., *Rheumatoid Arthritis*, 1st edition. Philadelphia: Mosby 2009:15–22.

14. Gonzalez A, Maradit Kremers H, Crowson CS, et al. The widening mortality gap between rheumatoid arthritis patients and the general population. *Arthritis Rheum* 2007;56(11):3583–7.

15. Gonzalez A, Icen M, Kremers HM, et al. Mortality trends in rheumatoid arthritis: The role of rheumatoid factor. *J Rheumatol* 2008;35(6):1009–1014.

16. Elena Myasoedova and Sherine E. Gabriel "Cardiovascular disease in rheumatoid arthritis: a step forward. *Current Opinion in Rheumatology* 2010, 22:342–347.

Chapter 4

Pathogenesis

In rheumatoid arthritis (RA), the site of the initial inflammatory process is the synovial lining of diarthrodial joints,[1] where synovial fluid provides the nutrition for the articular cartilage and lubricates the cartilage surfaces. During the inflammatory process, the synovial tissue undergoes increased vascularization and infiltration by lymphocytes, plasma cells, and activated macrophages.[1] As the disease progresses, a pannus forms from the progressive overgrowth of this tissue as it covers the articular surface.[1]

Although the etiology and pathogenesis of RA have yet to be completely specified, a number of factors have been identified as contributing to the disease process. These factors include genetics, environmental sources, the interaction of genes and environment, and cellular abnormalities. Over the past two decades, our understanding of the molecular pathogenesis of RA has increased exponentially, thanks to important advances in the treatment of RA. Tumor necrosis factor (TNF), for example, has been identified as a proinflammatory cytokine activated in the synovium of RA patients,[2] leading to treatments such as etanercept (Enbrel), infliximab (Remicade), adalimumab (Humira), golimumab (Simponi), and certolizumab pegol (Cimzia) that directly inhibit the proinflammatory cytokines and/or interfere with their receptor binding.[2]

Genetics

Studies of families and of monozygotic and dizygotic twins confirm the presence of a genetic component to RA. In an effort to determine the magnitude of this genetic component, MacGregor et al. used quantitative methods to analyze the results from two of the largest twin studies (one from Finland and one from the United Kingdom) to estimate the extent to which RA can be explained by genetic variation.[3] Their analysis determined that approximately 60% of RA susceptibility risk is attributable to heritability.[3]

At the present stage of our knowledge, the two major genetic risk factors associated with RA are the shared epitope of the major histocompatibility complex (MHC) associated with the alleles within the HLA-DRB1 gene (4,5) and the non-MHC, non-HLA A allele PTPN22 R620W.[5] The frequency of the HLA allele in the normal population is quite diverse, whereas the same allele is preferentially expressed in the region of the HLA-DRB1 gene cluster in RA patients.[6] Estimates indicate that the risk for RA associated with the MHC region of the human genome is approximately 30%. [7–9] The magnitude of the genetic risk associated with PTPN22 is somewhat less than that associated with HLA-DRB1.[9] The presence of these polymorphisms in RA patients differs by ethnicity. For example, the PTPN22 allele is not present in East Asians.[10]

Separately, the presence of HLA-DRB1 and PTPN22 R620W are each associated with an increased risk for the development of anti-cyclic citrullinated peptide (CCP)-positive RA.[5] In addition to the individual association of each of these polymorphisms with anti-CCP positive RA, an interaction exists between the two that is also associated with anti-CCP positive RA.[5]

Environmental Risk Factors

Research into the association between environmental risk factors and RA is relatively recent, with the majority of findings having been published during the past 25 years. Environmental risk factors have been studied principally in conjunction with disease onset, with relatively few studies examining the association between environmental risk on disease progression and comorbidities.[11]

The primary known environmental risk factor for RA is cigarette smoking,[12] a serendipitous finding resulting from a study of the possible association between oral contraceptive use and RA. Smoking increases the risk of developing seropositive, but not seronegative, RA.[13] The risk of developing seropositive RA is dose-dependent and increases with the number of years ever smoked.[13] Former smokers remain at risk for RA for anywhere between 10 and 19 years after smoking cessation.[13]

Hart et al. observed that the prevalence of RA in the United States differs by geographical region, with higher prevalence rates in those regions with greater air pollution.[14] This finding, coupled with the association between smoking and local lung and systemic inflammation, led Hart et al. to hypothesize that inhaled particulate matter from traffic pollution might contribute to the risk of developing RA. They studied the relationship between proximity to the nearest road and incident RA among women enrolled in the Nurses Health Study. Proximity to the nearest road was used as a proxy for traffic pollution exposure. Results from this study indicate that there is a 31% increase in RA risk for women living within 50 meters of primary and secondary roads, compared to women living more than 200 meters from the same type of roads.[14]

Other investigations have explored the relationship between RA and alcohol use, birth weight, and early life hygiene. Data from two independent case–control studies of RA suggests that there may be a dose-dependent inverse risk associated with alcohol consumption and RA.[15] An analysis of women enrolled in the Nurses Health Study found that, when compared to women with an average birth weight, women with a higher birth weight (>4.54 kg) had a two-fold increased risk of adult onset RA.[16] Edwards[17] studied the early growth and early postnatal history of enrollees in the Hertfordshire Cohort Studies for potential associations with RA. Although there was no evidence for an association between early growth and RA, there was an association, among women only, between RA and having shared a bedroom during childhood,[17] the possibility being that proximity to another confers some amount of immunity.

A number of studies have examined the relationship between oral contraceptive pill (OCP) use and the risk of developing RA. Although the majority of these studies have shown that the use of OCPs confer a protective effect, others have failed to demonstrate an association.[18] Interestingly, though, an inverse relationship between OCP use and the presence of rheumatoid factor (RF) has been found in healthy women without RA, an association that held even after adjusting for age, education, and smoking.[18] This study suggests that the exogenous hormones found in oral contraceptives may have a role during the early stages of the immune dysregulation associated with RA.[18]

Pregnancy has been shown to confer a protective effect in women with established RA. On the other hand, there is some evidence linking nulliparity to an increased risk for susceptibility to RA. Spector et al. conducted a case–control study to examine the relationship between OCP use and parity in the development of RA. In addition to finding that nulliparity is a risk factor for the development of RA, they found a multiplicative relationship between nulliparity and OCP use, whereby nulliparous non-OCP users had a four-fold risk of RA when compared to parous OCP users.[19] One message here is that exogenous hormones, or even endogenous ones, may confer different risks depending on the age of the subject and perhaps the status of the immune system at different ages of the patient.

Various environmental risk factors, including mineral oils, silica, infections, blood transfusions, and dietary factors have been studied for their contribution to the risk of developing of RA. However, the evidence for the contribution for each of these potential risk factors is often conflicting and less definitive than the association between RA and smoking.[11,20]

Gene–Environment Interaction

Recently, a significant amount of research has focused on the interaction between smoking and the genetic risk inherent in the HLA DRB1 and the PTPN22 genes. Although the specific mechanism whereby smoking and genes interact has yet to be completely articulated, it appears that smoking promotes the citrullination of self proteins and, as such, may generate pathogenic autoantigen-driven responses.[21] Consistent with this thesis, several European studies support the presence of a gene–environment interaction between smoking and the HLA-DR SE genes for anticitrulline-positive RA, but not for anticitrulline-negative RA.[22–24] However, the finding of a gene–environment interaction for anti-CCP formation between shared epitope alleles was not substantiated in a study of three North American RA cohorts.[25] There is some evidence that a multiplicative gene–environment interaction between heavy smoking and PTPN22 contributes to RA risk.[26]

Molecular Pathogenesis

The mechanism of action by which RA is activated and by which progressive inflammation and damage occurs is a complex cellular interplay between several key cell types and processes. One of the fundamental elements in the initiation of the disease process is the abnormal presentation of self antigen by antigen-presenting cells (APC), such as B cells, dendritic cells, or macrophages,[2] which leads to the activation of autoreactive T lymphocytes.[27] As the disease progresses, the sublining of the synovium is infiltrated by T cells, B cells, macrophages, and plasma cells.[28] T cells, once activated, build up in the affected joint and secrete lymphokines such as interferon γ and interleukin-2,[2] as well as proinflammatory cytokines that are responsible for attracting and activating additional cells.[6] In addition to acting as APC, B cells produce RF and other autoantibodies, secrete proinflammatory cytokines such as tumor necrosis factor (TNF)-α, and activate T cells.[29] Macrophages, in addition to secreting cytokines, also stimulate synoviocytes to release enzymes, such as collagenases and proteases, that may lead to cartilage and bone damage.[6]

Several other cell types infiltrate and accumulate in the synovial membrane of RA patients via activated endothelial cells,[2] including synovial fibroblasts[29] and osteoclasts,[2] both responsible for bone degradation. Synovial fibroblasts contribute to cartilage and joint destruction through the expression of matrix-degrading enzymes, such as matrix metalloproteinases (MMPs),[30] and are activated by a variety of cytokines including TNF-α and interleukin-1.[30] The identification and understanding of this process has led to the development of several novel therapeutic strategies that target these cytokines.[30] Osteoclasts resorb bone matrix and are complemented by osteoblasts that produce bone matrix. Macrophage colony-stimulating factor (MCSF) and the receptor antagonist of NF-κB ligand (RANKL) are required for the growth and differentiation needed by osteoclasts to become fully developed.[31] An abnormal activation of osteoclasts leads to the bone destruction observed in RA patients,[32] in whom osteoclast formation in inflamed joints is produced by proinflammatory cytokines through their influence on RANKL expression.[31] Figure 4.1 represents a current model of the hypothesized pathogenesis of RA.

While Figure 4.1 represents one model of the pathogenesis of RA, researchers continue to vigorously pursue additional models to explain how the inflammatory mechanisms of RA may be inhibited. Two models in particular are undergoing current investigation: the JAK/STAT signaling pathway and the role of spleen tyrosine kinase (SyK) as a crucial cell signaling regulator.

JAKs, a family of cytoplasmic protein tyrosine kinases, have a significant influence in mediating inflammatory immune responses and their pharmacological properties are being examined in the treatment of inflammatory immune-mediated diseases.[33] CP-690,550 is a small molecule JAK antagonist currently being tested in clinical trials for the treatment of RA. In a phase IIa trial of 3 dosage levels (5 mg, 15 mg, 30 mg twice daily) of orally administered CP-690,550, Kremer et al report that compared to the placebo group, all three treatment groups receiving CP-690,550 achieved statistically significant and clinically meaningful improvements in disease activity.[34] Headache and nausea were the most common adverse events. Patients in all treatment arms had measurable increases in mean low-density lipoprotein cholesterol, high-density lipoprotein cholesterol, and mean serum creatinine levels.[34] A phase III 6-month, randomized, double-blind placebo-controlled study tested the efficacy, safety, and tolerability of 5 mg and 10 mg twice daily CP-690,550 (tasocitinib) and, consistent with the phase IIa trial, CP-690,550 demonstrated clinically significant efficacy.[35] No new safety signals were discovered.

The role of tyrosine kinase activity is being investigated for the way in which it activates receptor cells that release key inflammatory ingredients such as

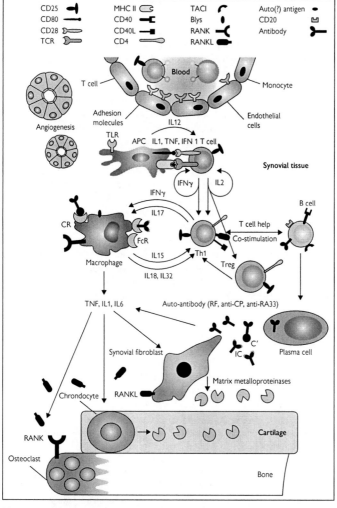

Figure 4.1 Current views on pathogenesis of rheumatoid arthritis. Arrows show some of many interactions in rheumatoid arthritis pathogenesis. Schematic depiction of events presumably occurring in synovial membrane, as well as articular cartilage and subchondral bone, which are surrounded by aggressive rheumatoid synovitis. Blys=B lymphocyte stimulator. C'=complement. CP=citrullinated peptide. CR=complement receptor. FcR=receptor for the Fc portion of IgG. IC= immune complex. IFN=interferon. IFN1=type 1 interferons. IL=interleukin. RF=rheumatoid factor. TACI=transmembrane activator and calciummodulator and cyclophilin ligand interactor. TCR=T-cell receptor. Th1=T-helper 1 cell. TLR=Toll-like receptor. Treg=regulatory T cell.

Reprinted from Lancet Vol 370, Smolen JS, Aletaha D, Koeller M et al. New therapies for treatment of rheumatoid arthritis, 1861–1874, 2007, with permission from Elsevier.

proinflammatory cytokines, MMPs, and lipid mediators of inflammation.[36] Of particular interest in this model is the spleen tyrosine kinase (Syk), an important regulator of cell signaling that is induced by cytokines or Fc receptors and has been discovered in the intimal lining of synovial tissue in RA patients.[37] Furthermore, in murine models, Syk inhibition suppressed synovial cytokines and cartilage oligomeric matrix protein (COMP) in serum.[38]

The effectiveness of R406, an inhibitor of SyK kinase, and its prodrug R788 have been studied as potential new therapeutic targets for the treatment of RA. There have been three clinical trials of the prodrug R788 that have produced mixed results. [36,39,40] A 12-week double-blind, placebo-controlled of twice-daily doses of 100 mg and 150 mg of R788 in RA patients proved superior to placebo in achieving significant clinical benefits.[36] A similar 6-month trial also yielded significant clinical benefits, although adverse events included diarrhea, hypertension, and neutropenia.[39] The third trial, a 3-month randomized, double-blind, placebo-controlled trial of R788 100 mg twice daily in RA patients who failed biologic treatment did not find significant differences between treatment and placebo groups in the primary endpoint of disease activity score, but did find significant differences between the groups in CRP level and synovitis score on MRI.[40] The results of these studies appear to indicate that at least 2 newly identified pathways might prove amenable as targets for orally administered agents. However, inhibition of these targets appears to produce a wide range of potentially undesirable side effects, the significance of which is currently under investigation.

References

1. Otero M, Goldring MB. Cells of the synovium in rheumatoid arthritis. Chondrocytes. *Arthritis Res Ther* 2007;9(5):220.

2. Smolen JS, Aletaha D, Koeller M, et al. New therapies for treatment of rheumatoid arthritis. *Lancet* 2007;370(9602):1861–1874.

3. MacGregor AJ, Snieder H, Rigby AS, et al. Characterizing the quantitative genetic contribution to rheumatoid arthritis using data from twins. *Arthritis Rheum* 2000;43(1):30–37.

4. Padyukov L, Silva C, Stolt P, et al. A gene–environment interaction between smoking and shared epitope genes in HLA-DR provides a high risk of seropositive rheumatoid arthritis. *Arthritis Rheum* 2004;50(10):3085–3092.

5. Källberg H, Padyukov L, Plenge RM, et al. Gene–gene and gene–environment interactions involving HLA-DRB1, PTPN22, and smoking in two subsets of rheumatoid arthritis. *Am J Hum Genet* 2007;80(5):867–875.

6. VanderBorght A, Geusens P, Raus J, Stinissen P. The autoimmune pathogenesis of rheumatoid arthritis: Role of autoreactive T cells and new immunotherapies. *Semin Arthritis Rheum* 2001;31(3):160–175.

7. Deighton CM, Walker DJ, Griffiths ID, Roberts DF. The contribution of HLA to rheumatoid arthritis. *Clin Genet* 1989;36(3):178–182.

8. Hasstedt SJ, Clegg DO, Ingles L, Ward RH. HLA-linked rheumatoid arthritis. *Am J Hum Genet* 1994;55(4):738–746.

9. Rigby AS, Silman AJ, Voelm L, et al. Investigating the HLA component in rheumatoid arthritis: an additive (dominant) mode of inheritance is rejected, a recessive mode is preferred. *Genet Epidemiol* 1991;8(3):153–175.

10. Plenge RM. The genetic basis of rheumatoid arthritis. In Hochberg MC, et al., eds., *Rheumatoid Arthritis*, 1st edition. Philadelphia: Mosby 2009:23–27.

11. Klareskog L, Rönnelid J, Alfredsson L. Environmental risk factors for rheumatoid arthritis. In Hochberg MC, et al., eds., *Rheumatoid Arthritis*, 1st edition. Philadelphia: Mosby 2009:28–34.

12. Klareskog L, Padyukov L, Alfredsson L. Smoking as a trigger for inflammatory rheumatic diseases. *Curr Opin Rheumatol* 2007;19(1):49–54.

13. Stolt P, Bengtsson C, Nordmark B, et al. Quantification of the influence of cigarette smoking on rheumatoid arthritis: Results from a population based case-control study, using incident cases. *Ann Rheum Dis* 2003;62(9):835–841.

14. Hart JE, Laden F, Puett RC, et al. Exposure to traffic pollution and increased risk of rheumatoid arthritis. *Environ Health Perspect* 2009;117(7):1065–1069.

15. Källberg H, Jacobsen S, Bengtsson C, et al. Alcohol consumption is associated with decreased risk of rheumatoid arthritis: Results from two Scandinavian case-control studies. *Ann Rheum Dis* 2009;68(2):222–227.

16. Mandl LA, Costenbader KH, Simard JF, Karlson EW. Is birthweight associated with risk of rheumatoid arthritis? Data from a large cohort study. *Ann Rheum Dis* 2009;68(4):514–518.

17. Edwards CJ, Goswami R, Goswami P, et al. Growth and infectious exposure during infancy and the risk of rheumatoid factor in adult life. *Ann Rheum Dis* 2006;65(3):401–404.

18. Bhatia SS, Majka DS, Kittelson JM, et al. Rheumatoid factor seropositivity is inversely associated with oral contraceptive use in women without rheumatoid arthritis. *Ann Rheum Dis* 2007;66(2):267–269.

19. Spector TD, Roman E, Silman AJ. The pill, parity, and rheumatoid arthritis. *Arthritis Rheum* 1990;33(6):782–789.

20. Hochberg MC, Oliver JE, Silman AJ. Risk factors for rheumatoid arthritis: Other nongenetic host factors. In Hochberg MC, et al., eds., *Rheumatoid Arthritis*, 1st edition. Philadelphia: Mosby 2009:35–40.

21. McInnes IB, Schett G. Cytokines in the pathogenesis of rheumatoid arthritis. *Nat Rev Immunol* 2007;7(6):429–442.

22. Klareskog L, Stolt P, Lundberg K, et al. A new model for an etiology of rheumatoid arthritis: Smoking may trigger HLA-DR (shared epitope)-restricted immune reactions to autoantigens modified by citrullination. *Arthritis Rheum* 2006;54(1):38–46.

23. Pedersen M, Jacobsen S, Garred P, et al. Strong combined gene–environment effects in anti-cyclic citrullinated peptide-positive rheumatoid arthritis. *Arthritis Rheum* 2007;56(5):1446–1453.

24. Linn-Rasker SP, van der Helm-van Mil AH, van Gaalen FA, et al. Smoking is a risk factor for anti-CCP antibodies only in rheumatoid arthritis patients who carry HLA-DRB1 shared epitope alleles. *Ann Rheum Dis* 2006;65(3):366–371.

25. Lee HS, Irigoyen P, Kern M, et al. Interaction between smoking, the shared epitope, and anti-cyclic citrullinated peptide: A mixed picture in three large North American rheumatoid arthritis cohorts. *Arthritis Rheum* 2007;56(6):1745–1753.

26. Costenbader KH, Chang S-C, DeVivo I, et al. Genetic polymorphisms in *PTPN22*, *PADI-4*, and *CTLA-4* and risk for rheumatoid arthritis in two longitudinal cohort studies: Evidence of gene–environment interactions with heavy cigarette smoking. *Arthritis Res Ther* 2008,10(3):R52. Epub 2008 May 7.

27. Thomas R, MacDonald KP, Pettit A, et al. Dendritic cells and the pathogenesis of rheumatoid arthritis. *J Leukoc Biol* 1999;66(2):286–292.

28. Lee DM, Weinblatt ME. Rheumatoid arthritis. *Lancet* 2001;358(9285):903–911.

29. Panayi GS. B cells: A fundamental role in the pathogenesis of rheumatoid arthritis? *Rheumatology* 2005;44(Suppl. 2):ii3-ii7.

30. Pap T, Müller-Ladner U, Gay RE, Gay S. Fibroblast biology. Role of synovial fibroblasts in the pathogenesis of rheumatoid arthritis. *Arthritis Res* 2000;2(5):361–367.

31. Schett G, Redlich K. Osteoclasts and Osteoblasts. In Hochberg MC, et al., eds., *Rheumatoid Arthritis,* 1st edition. Philadelphia: Mosby 2009:163–167.

32. Sato K, Takayanagi H. Osteoclasts, rheumatoid arthritis, and osteoimmunology. *Curr Opin Rheumatol* 2006;18(4):419–426.

33. Ghoreschi K, Jesson MI, Li X, et al. Modulation of innate and adaptive immune responses by tofacitinib (CP-690,550). *J Immunol* 2011;186(7):4234–4243.

34. Kremer JM, Bloom BJ, Breedveld FC, et al. The safety and efficacy of a JAK inhibitor in patients with active rheumatoid arthritis. *Arthritis Rheum* 2009;60(7):1895–1905.

35. Fleischmann RM, Kremer JM, Cush JJ, et al. Phase 3 study of oral JAK inhibitor tasocitinib (CP-690,550) monotherapy in patients with active rheumatoid arthritis. *Arthritis Rheum* 2010;62(Suppl 10):L8.

36. Weinblatt ME, Kavanaugh A, Burgos-Vargas R, et al. Treatment of rheumatoid arthritis with a Syk kinase inhibitor: a twelve-week randomized, placebo-controlled trial. *Arthritis Rheum* 2008;58(11):3309–3318.

37. Cha HS, Boyle DL, Inoue T, et al. A novel spleen tyrosine kinase inhibitor blocks c-Jun N-terminal kinase-mediated gene expression in synoviocytes. *J Pharmacol Exp Ther* 2006;317(2):571–578.

38. Pine PR, Chang B, Schoettler N, et al. Inflammation and bone erosion are suppressed in models of rheumatoid arthritis following treatment with a novel Syk inhibitor. *Clin Immunol* 2007;124(3):244–257.

39. Weinblatt ME, Kavanaugh A, Genovese MC, et al. An oral spleen tyrosine kinase (Syk) inhibitor for rheumatoid arthritis. *N Engl J Med* 2010;363(14):1303–1312.

40. Genovese MC, Kavanaugh A, Weinblatt ME, et al. A three-month randomized, placebo-controlled, phase II study in patients with active rheumatoid arthritis that did not respond to biologic agents. *Arthritis Rheum* 2011;63(2):337–345.

Chapter 5

Clinical Signs and Symptoms

Rheumatoid arthritis (RA) is not a homogeneous condition. It is, rather, a heterogeneous disease that differs among patients in clinical manifestations and outcome, with some patients experiencing a mild nonerosive form while others experience an aggressive and persistent disease with severe articular damage.[1] The onset of RA is equally heterogeneous. Seventy percent of patients present with a slow, insidious onset; 20% with an intermediate onset; and the remaining 10% with a sudden acute onset.[2] Irrespective of the type of onset, physiologic changes may occur in the synovial environment even during the asymptomatic phase of the disease.[3] There is also strong evidence that joint damage occurs early in the course of RA,[3] although damage may continue to occur for up to 20 years following disease onset.[2]

The signs and symptoms most commonly associated with RA are pain, swelling, and morning stiffness in the peripheral joints. Joint swelling may begin only in a few joints, but ultimately is typically symmetric in its established form, and initially occurs in the upper extremities in over half of patients.[2] No laboratory tests exist to definitively prove the diagnosis of RA.[4] However, abnormal values in tests for systemic inflammation, such as erythrocyte sedimentation rate, other acute-phase proteins, and plasma viscosity are helpful diagnostic markers.[4] Structural damage is primarily determined with radiography,[3] although magnetic resonance imaging and ultrasound may be used to complement and even anticipate radiographic findings.

Disease progression is variable, and the course of RA may be cyclic or unrelentingly active.[5] Erosive damage is seen within 3 months of disease onset in between 10% and 26% of patients and, by 2 years, 75% of RA patients exhibit erosive joint damage.[1] Although it is impossible to predict the course of RA in any given patient, the presence of IgM rheumatoid factor (RF); anti-cyclic citrullinated peptide (CCP) antibodies, which confer an increased likelihood of damage in seropositive patients;[2] C-reactive protein (CRP); human leukocyte antigen (HLA) shared epitope (SE); and baseline radiographic damage are associated with disease progression.[1] Additionally, patterns of joint complaints may also serve as markers of disease progression. For example, younger patients with metacarpophalangeal (MCP) II, III, IV, and V involvement tend to have a more benign disease process than older, seropositive patients with shoulder, elbow, wrist, and knee complaints.[2] However, in an individual patient, these clinical phenotypes are insufficient to predict an exact prognosis.

Variations on classic seropositive RA include seronegative RA, present in an estimated 15%–20% of patients, and palindromic rheumatism. Despite the absence of RF, many of these seronegative patients eventually meet the criteria for established RA.[2] Patients with palindromic rheumatism experience acute, recurrent palindromic attacks of oligoarticular arthritis concurrent with peri- and para-articular tissue inflammation, with nodules present in some cases.[2] Among this population, about 50% of patients have a favorable prognosis and experience no bone or cartilage destructions, whereas the remaining 50% convert to typical RA with RF positivity.[2]

It is imperative to diagnosis RA as soon as possible and to initiate disease-modifying antirheumatic drug (DMARD) treatment immediately to slow disease progression and destruction, and to improve patient outcomes and quality of life.[3] Primary care physicians should refer patients to a rheumatologist as soon as a diagnosis of RA is suspected or made. This referral is made primarily to (a) confirm the diagnosis (as well as rule out other conditions), (b) establish prognostic factors for disease outcome, (c) determine a drug management program that outlines risk and benefit for that individual patient, and (d) solidify the relationship between the health care providers managing that patient so that a team approach can be utilized.

Clinical Features

Articular and Periarticular Manifestations

Typical signs and symptoms, clinical features, and radiographic findings for the articular and periarticular manifestations of RA in the upper and lower extremities are shown in Table 5.1.

Spine and Axial Joints

The introduction of new therapies and early, more aggressive treatment of RA patients have resulted in a decrease in the number of patients who experience complications from cervical spine abnormalities.[6] Moreover, the incidence and prevalence of cervical spine abnormalities is small relative to the frequency with which proximal interphalangeal (PIP) joints, MCP joints of the hands and wrists, and metatarsophalangeal (MTP) joints of the feet, ankles, and shoulders are affected. Among the common cervical spine abnormalities observed in RA patients with longstanding disease are atlantoaxial subluxation (the loss of ligamentous stability between atlas and axis), basilar invagination (the result of the odontoid migrating upward), and subaxial subluxation (occurring as a result of the destruction of the facet joints, interspinous ligaments, and discovertebral junctions below the atlantoaxial segment). Like cervical spine abnormalities, deformities of the thoracolumbar and sacral joints appear infrequently in RA patients.

It is common for RA patients to experience signs and symptoms in the sternoclavicular, manubriosternal, temporomandibular, and cricoarytenoid joints. Although clinical evidence appears in only 10% of RA patients, approximately 70% patients with erosive RA experience pain and swelling from sternoclavicular and manubriosternal articulations.[7] The more severe and prolonged the disease duration, the more likely it is that temporomandibular joint (TMJ) symptoms will occur.[8] Involvement of the cricoarytenoid joint rarely results in complications, but may be present in between 26% and 86% of RA patients.[9,10]

Table 5.1 Upper and Lower Extremity Articular and Periarticular Manifestations of Rheumatoid Arthritis (RA)

Location	Percent of Patients Affected	Signs and Symptoms	Clinical Exam	Radiographic Findings
Upper Extremity				
Hand	• 55% of RA patients experience tenderness, warmth, and swelling along the flexor or extensor digital tendons. • MCP joints are usually the "calling card" of patients with RA and distinguish this disease clinically from osteoarthritis even in its inflammatory forms.	• Pain and swelling of the MCP and PIP joints, usually symmetric. • Pain and stiffness worse in the morning. • Tendon ruptures presenting as painless, sudden loss of extension or flexion. • With ongoing inflammation, evidence of clinical hypertrophy of the synovial lining and inflammation of periarticular structures.	• Warm, erythematous joints with effusions. • Soft tissue swelling around the MCP and PIP joints. • Decreased grip strength. • Synovial thickening can be detected on physical exam by feeling a bogginess of the joint on palpation. • In later stages of RA, there are anatomic disruptions of the integrity of the joint surfaces, ligaments, and tendons that cause visible joint deformities such as the boutonniere and swan neck deformities.	• Joint space narrowing of MCP and PIP joints. • Soft tissue swelling related to joint effusion, synovitis, and periarticular edema.
Wrist	• Up to 50% of patients experience wrist involvement in the first two years from disease onset.[11] • Up to 75% of patients will experience wrist involvement during the course of the disease.[12]	• Pain, swelling, limited range of motion, usually symmetric. • Pain and stiffness worse in the morning. • Pain on the radial aspect of the wrist that may radiate proximally caused by tenosynovitis. • Loss of wrist extension. • Decreased sensation with numbness and tingling especially in the night-time hours.	• Swelling is most prominent dorsally as well as over the ulnar styloid, and a typical feature is often visible swelling and rope-like thickening of the extensor carpi ulnaris tendon sheath. • Ongoing inflammation can lead to erosions, tenosynovitis, and nerve compression. • Chronic inflammation at the wrist leads to deformities, loss of function, and bony attrition, affecting adjacent tendons that may result in tendon rupture.	• Progression of carpal involvement measured by cartilage loss and bone compaction at the radial to lunate, lunate to capitate, and capitate to third metacarpal articulations. • Radial deviation at the wrist can be readily seen on a PA radiograph when more than half of the lunate articular surface is no longer articulating with the radius.

(continued)

Table 5.1 Continued

Location	Percent of Patients Affected	Signs and Symptoms	Clinical Exam	Radiographic Findings
Elbow	• Incidence of mild erosions: 33%. • Incidence of severe erosions: 18%.	• Loss of full extension at the elbow, of which patients may be unaware due to compensatory function by wrists and shoulders.	• Mild flexion contractures and nodule formation on the extensor surface of the elbow that may lead to cortical bone erosions in the underlying ulna and radius and appear like scalloped defects. • With continued inflammation, the valgus angulation can become three times greater than normal with severe flexion contractures leading to functional disability. • Erosions are most observed on the capitellum, the lateral epicondyle, and the olecranon.	• Soft tissue changes are seen with joint effusions displacing the anterior and posterior fat pads. • Initial positional changes include an anterior, anterolateral, or ventral subluxation of the radial head in relation to the capitellum of the humerus. • Late radiographic changes of joint destruction of the elbow are narrowing of the humeroradial and humeroulnar joint spaces, and marked bone destruction of both the humerus and the olecranon bones at their articulating surfaces.
Shoulder	• Incidence of mild erosions: 27%. • Incidence of severe erosions: 21%. • 55% of seropositive RA patients develop erosions of the glenohumeral joints within 15 years of disease onset.	• Shoulder pain and stiffness. • Decreased range of motion. • Difficulty sleeping.	• Limited abduction and external rotation of the affected arm. • Shoulder joint, rotator cuff muscles, and shoulder bursa may be affected. • Synovitis may present with an anterior effusion resembling a mass. • Inflammation can progress to destruction of the rotator cuff muscles, superior subluxation of the humeral head, and extension of the pannus into the glenohumeral joint.	• Radiographic findings are typically absent in early RA shoulder involvement in spite of a great deal of pain and limited mobility of the joint. • A late finding on radiography is glenohumeral joint space narrowing, indicating more marked erosive destruction.

| | | | • A very late and uncommon finding is rupture of the long head of the biceps tendon presenting as a soft tissue mass in the upper arm. |
| | | • With continued chronic inflammation, weakening of the rotator cuff muscles will cause superior subluxation of the humeral head.
• Acromioclavicular joint damage is commonly seen and correlates well with glenohumeral joint destruction. | |

Lower Extremity

| Foot and Ankle | • 90% of RA patients will experience foot and ankle manifestations during the course of their disease. | • Pain on weight-bearing movement and walking.
• Swelling of the feet may necessitate an increase in shoe size.
• Forefoot is the most common painful area.
• Heel pain is uncommon.
• Patients may complain of paresthesias if synovitis compresses the tarsal tunnel where the posterior tibial nerve runs. | • Swelling in the synovium and soft tissues of the metatarsal-phalangeal joints may cause the metatarsal heads to splay laterally so that a light shining between the toes can be seen.
• A slight squeeze across the MTP joints may prove very tender.
• Hallux valgus is present when the first metatarsal and the base of the first phalange are at an angle greater than 20 degrees.
• The hind foot structures (ankle and subtalar joints) are typically affected; grasping the hind foot and inverting it at the level of the ankle will cause stress pain across the subtalar joint. | • Early radiograph changes include periarticular osteopenia and soft tissue swelling.
• The forefoot usually displays the earliest changes with the lateral fifth metatarsal head first to show an erosion as well as the medial side of the proximal interphalangeal joint of the great toe.
• Diffuse joint space narrowing of the ankle and tarsal articulations may also be observed.
• With continued inflammation, the AP radiography may show proximal phalanges end-on, or the "gun-barrel sign." |

(continued)

Table 5.1 Continued

Location	Percent of Patients Affected	Signs and Symptoms	Clinical Exam	Radiographic Findings
Knee	• 70% to 80% of RA patients will experience knee involvement (4).	• Pain associated with weight bearing and restriction of movement of the knee. • Weakness, contractures, and difficulty walking occur with persistent inflammation.	• Synovial hypertrophy can be palpated in the supra-patellar pouch and alongside the inferior margins of the patella. • Effusions may be observed by patellar tap ("ballottement") or the bulge sign.	• Joint effusion with enlargement of the suprapatellar bursa on lateral films. • Narrowing of medial and lateral knee compartments on weight bearing films as well as bare area erosions, and valgus or varus deformities may occur as the disease progresses. • Popliteal or Baker's cysts.
Hip	• 10% in patients with disease duration less than 10 years. • 40% in patients with disease duration more than 10 years.	• Stiffness. • Groin pain or medial knee pain that is referred from the hip.	• Limited range of motion (by pain) may be demonstrated in all directions but with rotation primarily affected in the early stages.	• Diffuse joint space narrowing with erosions of the femoral head and neck. • Osteonecrosis or avascular necrosis. • Protrusio deformities can take place in very late stage RA hip involvement.

Extra-articular Features

Extra-articular RA (ExRA) manifestations may attack any of the major organ systems: cardiovascular, pulmonary, ocular, neurologic, skin, hematologic, renal, and hepatic.[4] Table 5.2 outlines ExRA manifestations by organ system.

The incidence and prevalence of any given ExRA manifestation is variable. Subcutaneous rheumatoid nodules are the most frequent ExRA manifestation, with an estimated 30% of all patients developing rheumatoid nodules at some point in their lifetime.[13] In one of the few community-based studies of the incidence of RA, the most common ExRA manifestations were rheumatoid nodules, secondary Sjögren's syndrome, and pulmonary fibrosis.[14]

Physicians treating RA patients should be alert to the presence of ExRA manifestations. Patients with ExRA manifestations may present with constitutional symptoms, such as weight loss, fatigue, low-grade fever, and elevated levels of inflammatory biomarkers.[4,15] RA patients, particularly current smokers and those with early disability, are particularly at risk for developing extra-articular RA,[14] and severe ExRA complications occur primarily in RF-seropositive patients.[16]

Table 5.2 Extra-articular RA Manifestations by Organ System[1]

Constitutional symptoms
 Fever
 Asthenia
 Weight loss
 Malaise
 Anorexia

Rheumatoid nodules
 Subcutaneous
 Lung parenchymal

Cardiovascular
 Vasculitis (coronary arteritis)
 Pericardial inflammation and effusion
 Myocarditis
 Mitral valve disease
 Conduction defects

Pulmonary
 Pleural effusions
 Pulmonary nodules
 Interstitial fibrosis
 Pneumonitis
 Arteritis

Ocular
 Keratoconjunctivitis sicca
 Episcleritis
 Scleritis
 Conjunctivits

Table 5.2 Continued

Neurologic
  Compression neuropathy (such as carpal tunnel syndrome)
  Mononeuritis multiplex
  Cervical myelopathy
  Central nervous system disease (stroke, seizure, hemorrhage,
  encephalopathy, meningitis)

Skin
  Distal leg ulcers
  Palmar erythema
  Cutaneous vasculitis

Hematologic
  Anemia
  Thrombocytosis
  Granulocytopenia
  Eosynophilia
  Cryoglobulinemia
  Hyperviscosity

Renal
  Glomerulonephritis
  Vasculitis
  Secondary amyloidosis

Hepatic
  Elevated liver enzymes

1 Reprinted from European Journal of Radiology Vol 27, Grassi W, DeAngelis R, Lamanna G, Cervini C. The clinical features of rheumatoid arthritis, S18-S24, 1998 with permission from Elsevier.

References

1. Soubrier M, Dougados M. How to assess early rheumatoid arthritis in daily clinical practice. *Best Pract Res Clin Rheumatol* 2005;19(1):73–89.

2. Posalski J, Weisman MH. Articular and periarticular manifestations of established rheumatoid arthritis. In Hochberg MC, et al., eds., *Rheumatoid Arthritis*, 1st edition. Philadelphia: Mosby 2009:49–61.

3. Emery P, Breedveld FC, Dougados M, et al. Early referral recommendation for newly diagnosed rheumatoid arthritis: Evidence-based development of a clinical guide. *Ann Rheum Dis* 2002;61(4):290–297.

4. Grassi W, DeAngelis R, Lamanna G, Cervini C. The clinical features of rheumatoid arthritis. *Eur J Radiol* 1998;27 Suppl 1:S18–24.

5. Smolen JS, Aletaha D, Grisar J, et al. The need for prognosticators in rheumatoid arthritis. Biological and clinical markers: where are we now? *Arthritis Res Ther* 2008;10(3):208.

6. van Eijk IC, Nielen MM, van Soesbergen RM, et al. Cervical spine involvement is rare in early arthritis. *Ann Rheum Dis* 2006;65(7):973–974.

7. Khong TK, Rooney PJ. Manubriosternal joint subluxation in rheumatoid arthritis. *J Rheumatol* 1982;9(5):712–715.

8. Goupille P, Fouquet B, Goga D, et al. The temporomandibular joint in rheumatoid arthritis: Correlations between clinical and tomographic features. *J Dent* 1993;21(3):141–146.

9. Kolman J, Morris I. Cricoarytenoid arthritis: A cause of acute upper airway obstruction in rheumatoid arthritis. *Can J Anaesth* 2002;49(7):729–732.

10. Chen JJ, Branstetter BF, Myers EN. Cricoarytenoid rheumatoid arthritis: An important consideration in aggressive lesions of the larynx. *Am J Neuroradiol* 2005;26(4):970–972.

11. Trieb K. Treatment of the wrist in rheumatoid arthritis. *J Hand Surg* 2008;33(1):113–123.

12. Ilan DI, Retting ME. Rheumatoid arthritis of the wrist. *Bull Hosp Joint Dis* 2003;61(3–4):179–185.

13. Nyhäll-Wahlin B, Jacobsson LT, Petersson IF, et al. Smoking is a strong risk factor for rheumatoid nodules in early rheumatoid arthritis. *Ann Rheum Dis* 2006;65(5):601–606.

14. Turesson C, O'Fallon WM, Crowson CS, et al. Extra-articular disease manifestations in rheumatoid arthritis: Incidence trends and risk factors over 46 years. *Ann Rheum Dis* 2003;62(8):722–727.

15. Turesson C, Matteson EL. Clinical features of rheumatoid arthritis: Extraarticular manifestations. In Hochberg MC, et al., eds., *Rheumatoid Arthritis*, 1st edition. Philadelphia: Mosby 2009:35–40.

16. Voskuyl AE, Zwinderman AH, Westedt ML, et al. Factors associated with the development of rheumatoid vasculitis: Results of a case control study. *Ann Rheum Dis* 1996;55(3):190–192.

Chapter 6

Comorbidities and Rheumatoid Arthritis

Several comorbidities and extra-articular manifestations of rheumatoid arthritis (RA) require special attention due to their particularly devastating effects. Linkages between RA and other diseases have been hypothesized and continue to be refined as our understanding of RA, its pathogenesis, and genetic basis continues to evolve. New research indicates that the inflammation common to atherosclerosis and RA is associated with an increased prevalence of ischemic heart disease (IHD) in RA patients. Pulmonary disease, particularly interstitial lung disease (ILD), shares several common lymphocyte subpopulations with key pathogenetic features of RA. Innovative new genetics research has identified common genetic susceptibility loci for the co-occurrence of RA and type 1 diabetes. Ironically, obesity, a risk factor for heart disease, diabetes, and hypertension, has a protective effect in patients with RA.

Cardiovascular Disease

The leading cause of death in RA patients is cardiovascular disease (CVD).[1-3] There is overwhelming evidence that the prevalence of cardiovascular morbidity and mortality is consistently higher in RA patients compared to the general population. For example, a recent study of a population-based incidence cohort using patients from the Rochester Epidemiology Project reported a >10% risk of CVD within 10 years of RA diagnosis among more than half of patients aged 50–59 years and among all patients >60 years.[4] A meta-analysis of 24 published studies covering a total of 111,758 patients with 22,927 cardiovascular events noted a 50% increase in the risk of CVD mortality in RA patients compared to the general population.[5]

Traditional cardiovascular risk factors do not sufficiently explain the excess risk of CVD among RA patients,[2] and current avenues of research are directed toward explaining the causes of this excess risk. One promising area of research focuses on the inflammatory process common to both atherosclerosis and RA. Inflammation plays a key role in the pathogenesis of atherosclerosis in the general population,[6] and the question arises as to whether the inflammation seen in RA patients accelerates the inflammatory process for atherosclerosis, thereby leading to excess cardiovascular risk. The same proinflammatory cytokines, such as interleukin (IL)-1α, IL-1β, IL-6, and tumor necrosis factor (TNF)-α, that drive the inflammatory process in RA are similarly implicated in the pathogenesis of atherosclerosis,[7-11] as are T-cell and mast cell activation.[9] It is hypothesized that the release of these proinflammatory cytokines may increase selected proatherogenic functions of other organs and tissue, such as the liver, adipose tissue, skeletal muscle, and vascular endothelium, eventually leading to insulin resistance, dyslipidemia, and endothelial activation.[9] Figure 6.1 illustrates how these mediators contribute to atherogenesis.

Increased C-reactive protein serum levels, another marker of the inflammatory process in RA patients, have also been implicated in the acceleration of atherosclerosis, as have CD40 ligand, IL-20, monocyte chemotactic protein (MCP)-1, fractalkine, and matrix metalloproteinase (MMP)-9.[10] The atherogenic side effects of medications used to treat RA and the chronic systemic inflammation sustained by the vascular endothelium may also contribute to the acceleration or exacerbation of atherogenesis in RA.[2]

Indirect evidence for accelerated atherosclerosis in RA patients comes primarily from studies measuring carotid artery intima–media thickness (IMT) and carotid artery plaque, both surrogate markers for coronary atherosclerosis. [6,11,12] Carotid IMT measurement is the weaker of these two indicators, due to the fact that it may also detect the presence of other aspects of vascular disease.[12] Hannawi et al. compared carotid IMT and carotid atherosclerotic plaque in patients with early RA. Compared to matched controls, patients with RA had significantly higher average carotid IMT values and increased plaque (0.58 ± 0.09 mm vs. 0.64 ± 0.13 mm, respectively; $p = 0.03$).[13] Gonazalez-Juanety et al. measured carotid IMT in patients with established RA and reported that, compared to matched controls, patients with RA had greater carotid IMT values (0.699 ± 0.129 mm vs. 0.779 ± 0.164 mm, respectively; $p = 0.010$).[11] In the

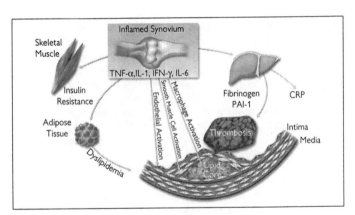

Figure 6.1 Diagram depicting the inflammatory pathways by which mediators of synovitis, including tumor necrosis factor (TNF)–α, may alter arterial biology and risk factors for atherosclerosis, including insulin resistance, dyslipidemia, fibrinogen, plasminogen activator inhibitor–1 (PAI-1), and heighten the production by the liver of the biomarker of inflammation C-reactive protein (CRP). IFN = interferon; IL = interleukin

Reprinted from The American Journal of Medicine, Vol 121, Libby P, Role of inflammation in atherosclerosis associated with rheumatoid arthritis, S21-S31, 2008, with permission from Elsevier.

same study, patients with RA without clinical evidence of atherosclerosis were compared to RA patients with documented carotid plaques. Rheumatoid arthritis patients with carotid plaques had significantly greater carotid IMT values than did patients without plaque.[11] Roman et al. measured the levels of carotid plaque in 98 RA patients and matched controls and found that RA patients had a three-fold increase in carotid atherosclerotic plaque (44% vs. 15%; p <0.001). Even after controlling for traditional risk factors, RA patients maintained higher levels of plaque than did their matched controls.[12] As an alternative to carotid IMT and plaque, Chung et al. measured coronary artery calcification in patients with early RA, established RA, and controls. Patients with established RA had significantly (p = 0.001) higher levels of coronary artery calcification (median 40.2, interquartile range 0–358.8) when compared to early RA patients (median 0, interquartile range 0–42.6) and controls (median 0, interquartile range 0–19.2). These associations remained significant even after adjusting for other cardiovascular risk factors.[14]

The presence of accelerated atherogenesis suggested by these and other studies is expressed in a higher incidence of ischemic cardiac pathologies in RA patients.[15] Indeed, increased morbidity and mortality in RA patients with IHD is well documented,[16–18] and the majority of the excess CVD risk in RA is partially attributable to IHD, with the remainder due to cerebrovascular accidents.[5] Concurrently, factors implicated in the pathogenesis of RA also serve as markers for increased risk of IHD in individuals both with and without RA. Using 767 patients from the Early RA Study, Mattey et al. sought to determine the contribution of the HLA-DRB1 shared epitope (SE) to morbidity and mortality in RA patients. Although the SE was not significantly related to overall mortality, two alleles on the SE, HLA–DRB1*0101/*0401 and 0404/*0404, were significantly associated with an increased risk of mortality from IHD.[19] In a study of 937 RA patients in Spain, López-Longo et al. determined that the presence of anti-cyclic citrullinated peptide (CCP) antibodies contribute to the development of IHD, irrespective of the quantity of the antibodies.[20] Interestingly, the presence of RF in men *without* RA was significantly associated with an increased risk for IHD, independent of traditional risk factors for IHD.[21] Although not specifically implicated as a risk factor for IHD, the increased prevalence of circulating CD4+CD28-null lymphocytes in RA patients has been linked to the possible progression of atherosclerosis.[6,17]

A model of this complex interplay of inflammatory markers, arising from the relationship between the atherosclerotic process and incipient RA, has yet to be fully articulated. However, physicians treating RA patients must be alert to the presence of these factors in order to identify patients who may benefit from early intervention to prevent or delay the onset and/or progression of CVD and IHD. Preliminary analyses indicate that treatment with methotrexate or TNF antagonists may reduce higher risk of CVD morbidity and mortality in RA patients by reducing inflammation and improving vascular function.[7,8,22]

Pulmonary Disease

Rheumatoid arthritis places patients at increased risk for lung disease, particularly interstitial lung disease (ILD). Interstitial lung disease involves the lung parenchyma and is comprised of a diverse set of noninfectious acute and chronic diseases.[23] Interstitial lung disease occurs in the general population as idiopathic interstitial pneumonia (IIP) and in patients with connective diseases.[23] Each form of ILD is pathologically distinct, with the most common subcategories being usual interstitial pneumonia (UIP) and nonspecific interstitial pneumonia (NSIP).[23] Rheumatoid arthritis is typically associated with UIP.[23,24] The American Thoracic Society and European Respiratory Society classify IIP into seven distinct entities based on clinical, radiologic, and histologic features.[25]

The prevalence of ILD in RA patients varies between 1% and 58%, depending on method of detection, disease criteria, and study population.[26] In a survey of a community-based RA cohort, in which the case definition relied on clinical diagnosis and the results of pulmonary function tests, the 10-year cumulative incidence of interstitial pneumonitis (IP) after diagnosis of RA was estimated to be 6% in patients diagnosed during the period 1975–1995.[27] Smoking is an independent risk factor for ILD, and ILD occurs more frequently in men.[28]

The onset of ILD is gradual and usually follows the diagnosis of RA by several years. However, ILD may occur simultaneously with or precede the onset of RA.[29] Patients with ILD may be asymptomatic for respiratory symptoms, have nonspecific clinical manifestations, or present with nonproductive cough and dyspnea upon exertion.[26] Pulmonary function tests, chest x-rays, high-resolution computed tomography (CT), and ^{99m}Tc-DTPA nuclear scans are used to differentially diagnosis ILD. Bronchoalveolar lavage (BAL) may be used to exclude other diagnoses such as infection, co-existing diseases, or malignancy.[29] A definitive diagnosis of ILD, however, requires a lung biopsy.[29]

The pathogenesis of ILD is unknown. Research being conducted to identify the immunopathophysiology of ILD in RA patients is focused on those cells involved in the pathogenesis of RA. These studies typically involve analysis of lung biopsy specimens from a very small number of patients with and without RA. For example, Atkins et al. studied B-cell lymphocytes from lung biopsies in patients with RA-associated IP ($N = 18$), idiopathic IP ($N = 21$), and controls ($N = 11$). The lung tissue specimens from patients with RA-associated UIP and idiopathic UIP differed from the lung tissue of normal controls in that the tissue specimens of the former were characterized by the presence of a significantly greater number of CD20+ B cells than were the tissue specimens of the latter.[30] Turesson et al. compared the lung biopsy specimens from patients with either nonspecific IP or usual IP to assess the presence of lymphocyte markers. Fifteen of the specimens had RA, 16 did not. There were a greater number CD4+ and CD8+ cells in the IP lesions in patients with RA compared to the lesions of patients with idiopathic IP.[31] Other studies have shown an increased prevalence of mast cells[32] and citrullination.[33] Although these studies demonstrate intriguing associations between a potentially similar pathogenesis in RA and ILD, they should not be considered proof that a causal relationship exists.

There is no known treatment for ILD. The outcome for RA patients with ILD is poor,[26] with some evidence suggesting that RA patients with NSIP have a better prognosis than those with UIP.[24] Treatment of RA patients with ILD is complicated by the fact that some of the medications used to treat RA may be associated with lung damage.[26]

Diabetes

Rheumatoid arthritis and type 1 diabetes (T1D) are among several autoimmune diseases that cluster together and may involve the presence of common genetic factors thought to predispose to autoimmunity.[34] Revolutionary advances in genome mapping have made it possible to begin to empirically enumerate possible disease susceptibility genes common to both RA and T1D. These advances have resulted in an ever-expanding body of evidence that supports the hypothesis that RA and T1D share common susceptibility genes. For example, Myerscough et al. tested five insulin-dependent diabetes mellitus (IDDM) susceptibility loci for evidence of linkage disequilibrium with RA in 255 RA families and found significant evidence for linkage disequilibrium with RA for the marker D6S446 at IDDM8. Although not statistically significant, the same study also found evidence for linkage disequilibrium of RA with two IDDM 5 markers (D6311 and D6S440).[34] In another example, Zhernakova et al. studied 350 patients with juvenile-onset T1D, 1,047 RA patients, and 929 controls to determine whether RA and T1D share a common risk locus. Results from this study demonstrate an association between T1D and RA in the *KIAA1109/Tenr/IL2/IL21* gene region.[35]

The PTPN22 gene[36] and the HLA class III genes[37] have also been implicated as genetic risk factors implicated in the co-occurrence of RA and T1D. Liao et al. demonstrated that, among T1D patients, the risk of developing RA may be partially attributable to the presence of the 620W PTPN22 allele. Notably, anti-CCP-positive but not anti-CCP-negative RA patients were at increased risk.[36] The SE of the major histocompatibility complex (MHC) associated with the alleles within the HLA-DRB1 gene have long been implicated in the pathogenesis of RA. Valdes et al. report that not only is the class III region of the MHC involved in T1D susceptibility, the strongest association was with a gene also involved in RA susceptibility—the rs2395106 that maps 5' to the NOTCH4 gene.[37] Refinements to the hypothesis that RA and T1D share common susceptibility genes continue to be published. It is possible that continued research in autoimmune genes will lead to the identification of effective treatments or even prevention strategies for both RA and T1D.

Obesity

Obesity is a significant risk factor for diabetes, hypertension, and cardiovascular disease. Of late, there has been reason to suspect that obesity may influence both the development and course of RA due to the inflammatory nature of adipose tissue. Results from studies that form the nucleus of this evolving scientific inquiry indicate that, although obesity is not associated with the development of RA,[38] it definitely influences disability,[39] joint destruction,[38,40] and mortality.[41] Surprisingly, in contrast to other conditions in which obesity exerts a negative influence, obesity appears to confer a protective effect in RA patients. Van der Helm-van Mil et al. assessed the impact of body mass index (BMI) on joint destruction in RA patients from the Leiden Early Arthritis Clinic (EAC) and RA patients from the BeSt study. At 3 years from diagnosis, BMI was independently and inversely associated with the level of joint destruction among anti-CCP-positive RA patients. The relationship between BMI and joint destruction did not hold for anti-CCP-negative RA patients.[38] In a study of 767 patients in Germany with early RA, Westhoff et al. also ascertained that BMI is inversely correlated with radiographic damage at baseline and 3-year follow-up. However, the negative relationship between BMI and joint damage was present only among RF-positive patients.[40]

The relationship between obesity and RA is complex and has yet to be fully explained. It is certainly possible that there may be competing effects. Although evidence demonstrates that BMI has a paradoxical effect on mortality, wherein patients with high BMI have lower mortality, the effect is mediated in part by comorbidity.[41] This finding, along with the results demonstrating that joint destruction occurs only among RF-positive and anti-CCP-positive RA patients, suggest that future research should focus on elucidating the mechanism of action of adipocytokines in this patient population.

References

1. Wolfe F, Mitchell DM, Sibley JT, et al. The mortality of rheumatoid arthritis. *Arthritis Rheum* 1994,37(4):481–494.

2. del Rincón I, Williams K, Stern MP, et al. High incidence of cardiovascular events in a rheumatoid arthritis cohort not explained by traditional cardiac risk factors. *Arthritis Rheum* 2001;44(12):2727–2745.

3. Gonzalez-Gay MA, Gonzalez-Juanatey C, Lopez-Diaz MJ, et al. HLA-DRB1 and persistent chronic inflammation contribute to cardiovascular events and cardiovascular mortality in patients with rheumatoid arthritis. *Arthritis Rheum* 2007;57(1):125–132.

4. Maradit-Kremers H, Crowson CS, Therneau TM, et al. High ten-year risk of cardiovascular disease in newly diagnosed rheumatoid arthritis patients: A population-based cohort study. *Arthritis Rheum* 2008;58(8):2268–2274.

5. Aviña-Zubieta JA, Choi HK, Sadatsafavi M, et al. Risk of cardiovascular mortality in patients with rheumatoid arthritis: A meta-analysis of observational studies. *Arthritis Rheum* 2008;59(12):1690–1697.

6. Warrington KJ, Kent PD, Frye RL, et al. Rheumatoid arthritis is an independent risk factor for multi-vessel coronary artery disease: A case control study. *Arthritis Res Ther* 2005;7(5):R984-R991.

7. Hürlimann D, Forster A, Noll G, et al. Anti-tumor necrosis factor-alpha treatment improves endothelial function in patients with rheumatoid arthritis. *Circulation* 2002;106(17):2184–2187.

8. Sattar N, McCarey DW, Capell H, McInnes IB. Explaining how "high-grade" systemic inflammation accelerates vascular risk in rheumatoid arthritis. *Circulation* 2003;108(24):2957–2963.

9. Libby P. Role of inflammation in atherosclerosis associated with rheumatoid arthritis. *Am J Med* 2008;121(10 Suppl 1):S21-S31.

10. Montecucco F, Mach F. Common inflammatory mediators orchestrate pathophysiological processes in rheumatoid arthritis and atherosclerosis. *Rheumatology* 2009;48(1):11–22.

11. Gonzalez-Juanatey C, Llorca J, Testa A, et al. Increased prevalence of severe subclinical atherosclerotic findings in long-term treated rheumatoid arthritis patients without clinically evident atherosclerotic disease. *Medicine* 2003;82(6):407–413.

12. Roman MJ, Moeller E, Davis A, et al. Preclinical carotid atherosclerosis in patients with rheumatoid arthritis. *Ann Intern Med* 2006;144(4):249–256.

13. Hannawi S, Haluska B, Marwick TH, Thomas R. Atherosclerotic disease is increased in recent-onset rheumatoid arthritis: A critical role for inflammation. *Arthritis Res Ther* 2007;9(6):R116.

14. Chung CP, Oeser A, Raggi P, et al. Increased coronary-artery atherosclerosis in rheumatoid arthritis. *Arthritis Rheum* 2005;52(10):3045–3053.

15. Douglas KM, Pace AV, Treharne GJ, et al. Excess recurrent cardiac events in rheumatoid arthritis patients with acute coronary syndrome. *Ann Rheum Dis* 2006;65(3):348–353.

16. Wallberg-Jonsson S, Öhman ML, Dahlqvist SR. Cardiovascular morbidity and mortality in patients with seropositive rheumatoid arthritis in northern Sweden. *J Rheumatol* 1997;24(3):445–451.

17. Gerli R, Schillaci G, Giordano A et al. CD4+CD28- T lymphocytes contribute to early atherosclerotic damage in rheumatoid arthritis patients. *Circulation* 2004;109(22):2744–2748.

18. Young A, Koduri G, Batley M, et al. Mortality in rheumatoid arthritis. Increased in the early course of disease, in ischaemic heart disease and in pulmonary fibrosis. *Rheumatology* 2007;46(2):350–357.

19. Mattey DL, Thomson W, Ollier WE, et al. Association of DRB1 shared epitope genotypes with early mortality in rheumatoid arthritis: Results of eighteen years of followup from the Early Rheumatoid Arthritis Study. *Arthritis Rheum* 2007;56(5):1408–1416.

20. Lopez-Longo FJ, Oliver-Miñarro O, de la Torre I, et al. Association between anti-cyclic citrullinated peptide and ischemic heart disease in patients with rheumatoid arthritis. *Arthritis Rheum* 2009;61(4):419–424.

21. Edwards CJ, Syddall H, Goswami R, et al. The autoantibody rheumatoid factor may be an independent factor for ischaemic heart disease in men. *Heart* 2007;93(10):1263–1267.

22. Carmona L, Descalzo MÁ, Perez-Pampin E, et al. All-cause and cause-specific mortality in rheumatoid arthritis are not greater than expected when treated with tumour necrosis factor antagonists. *Ann Rheum Dis* 2007;66(7):880–885.

23. Kocheril SV, Appleton BE, Somers EC, et al. Comparison of disease progression and mortality of connective tissue disease-related interstitial lung disease and idiopathic interstitial pneumonia. *Arthritis Rheum* 2005;53(4):549–557.

24. Lee H-K, Kim DS, Yoo B, et al. Histopathologic pattern and clinical features of rheumatoid arthritis-associated interstitial lung disease. *Chest* 2005;127(6):2019–2027.

25. American Thoracic Society, European Respiratory Society. American Thoracic Society/European Respiratory Society international multidisciplinary consensus classification of the idiopathic interstitial pneumonias: This joint statement of the American Thoracic Society (ATS), and the European Respiratory Society (ERS) was adopted by the ATS board of directors, June 2001 and by the ERS Executive Committee, June 2001 [published erratum appears in *Am J Respir Crit Care Med* 2002;166:426]. *Am J Respir Crit Care Med* 2002;165(2):277–304.

26. Nannini C, Ryu JH, Matteson EL. Lung disease in rheumatoid arthritis. *Curr Opin Rheumatol* 2008;20(3):340–346.

27. Turesson C, McClelland RL, Christianson TJ, Matteson EL. No decrease over time in the incidence of vasculitis or other extraarticular manifestations in rheumatoid arthritis: Results from a community-based study. *Arthritis Rheum* 2004;50(11):3729–3730.

28. Sundy JS, Jaffe GJ, McCallum. Extraarticular Disease. In St. Clair EM, Pisetsky DS, Haynes BF, eds., *Rheumatoid Arthritis*. Philadelphia: Lippincott Williams & Wilkins, 2004:483–495.

29. Kim DS. Interstitial lung disease in rheumatoid arthritis: recent advances. *Curr Opin Pulm Med* 2006;12(5):346–353.

30. Atkins SR, Turesson C, Myers JL, et al. Morphologic and quantitative assessment of CD20+ B cell infiltrates in rheumatoid arthritis-associated nonspecific interstitial pneumonia and usual interstitial pneumonia. *Arthritis Rheum* 2006;54(2):635–641.

31. Turesson C, Matteson EL, Colby TV, et al. Increased CD4+ T cell infiltrates in rheumatoid arthritis-associated interstitial pneumonitis compared with idiopathic interstitial pneumonitis. *Arthritis Rheum* 2005;52(1):73–79.

32. Atkins SR, Matteson EL, Myers JL, et al. Morphological and quantitative assessment of mast cells in rheumatoid arthritis associated non-specific interstitial pneumonia and usual interstitial pneumonia. *Ann Rheum Dis* 2006;65(5):677–680.

33. Bongartz T, Cantaert T, Atkins SR, et al. Citrullination in extra-articular manifestations of rheumatoid arthritis. *Rheumatology* 2007;46(1):70–75.

34. Myerscough A, John S, Barrett JH, et al. Linkage of rheumatoid arthritis to insulin-dependent diabetes mellitus loci: Evidence supporting a hypothesis for the existence of common autoimmune susceptibility loci. *Arthritis Rheum* 2000;43(12):2771–2775.

35. Zhernakova A, Alizadeh BZ, Bevova M, et al. Novel association in chromosome 4q27 region with rheumatoid arthritis and confirmation of type 1 diabetes point to a general risk locus for autoimmune diseases. *Am J Hum Genet* 2007;81(6):1284–1288.

36. Liao KP, Gunnarson M, Källberg H, et al. Specific association of type 1 diabetes mellitus with anti-cyclic citrullinated peptide-positive rheumatoid arthritis. *Arthritis Rheum* 2009;60(3):653–660.

37. Valdes AM, Thomson G; Type 1 Diabetes Genetics Consortium. Several loci in the HLA class III region are associated with T1D risk after adjusting for DRB1-DQB1. *Diabetes Obes Metab* 2009;11(Suppl 1):46–52.

38. van der Helm-van Mil AH, van der Kooij SM, Allaart CF, et al. A high body mass index has a protective effect on the amount of joint destruction in small joints in early rheumatoid arthritis. *Ann Rheum Dis* 2008;67(6):769–774.

39. Giles JT, Bartlett SJ, Andersen RE, et al. Association of body composition with disability in rheumatoid arthritis: Impact of appendicular fat and lean tissue mass. *Arthritis Rheum* 2008;59(10):1407–1415.

40. Westhoff G, Rau R, Zink A. Radiographic joint damage in early rheumatoid arthritis is highly dependent on body mass index. *Arthritis Rheum* 2007;56(11):3575–3582.

41. Escalante A, Haas RW, del Rincón I. Paradoxical effect of body mass index on survival in rheumatoid arthritis. *Arch Intern Med* 2005;165(14):1624–1629.

Chapter 7

Pregnancy

The course of rheumatoid arthritis (RA) is altered during pregnancy, with the majority of women experiencing some amelioration of symptoms and near complete remission in a minority of cases. Research to identify the molecular basis of the alleviation of RA symptoms in pregnant women continues to accumulate, although our understanding remains incomplete. Although the protective effect of pregnancy is annulled postpartum, pregnancy complications are not increased[1] and the prognosis for both the fetus and newborn is excellent.[1] The safety profile of anti-inflammatory agents, disease-modifying antirheumatic drugs (DMARDs), corticosteroids, and biologic agents must be considered prior to their use during pregnancy and during the postpartum period (i.e., breast-feeding).

Amelioration/Remission

One of the earliest observations of the remission of RA symptoms was noted in a patient with intercurrent jaundice and reported by Philip Showalter Hench in 1929.[2] Less than 10 years later, Hench observed that women with RA who became pregnant also experienced an amelioration of RA symptoms.[3] These recurring observations initiated Hench's pursuit to discover "an anti rheumatic substance X" responsible for the suppression of inflammation,[2] and eventually led to the discovery of cortisone, for which Hench and his colleagues were awarded the Nobel Prize in Medicine in 1950.[2] Although cortisone injections reduce inflammation in RA patients, the presence of increased serum cortisol is not responsible for symptom amelioration during pregnancy.[4]

Estimates of the percent of women who experience an amelioration or remission of symptoms during pregnancy vary from 54% to 86%.[1] Several factors account for these varying prevalence estimates, including the use of objective versus subjective measurements, whether RA was active prior to pregnancy, and treatment status prior to pregnancy.[5] Two large prospective studies provide additional details about the extent of symptom change during pregnancy. Barrett et al. prospectively followed 140 pregnant women with RA from their last trimester to 6 months postpartum. Symptom changes during the first two trimesters were based on patient recall, which may have introduced an element of bias to the study results. Among the study participants, there was a small statistically significant decline in Health Assessment Questionnaire (HAQ) scores from a median of 1.1 to a median of 0.9. Sixteen percent experienced complete remission, whereas 27% experienced considerable disability during pregnancy. Remission was greater among rheumatoid factor (RF)-negative women.[6] Based on the results of this study, Barrett et al. caution that symptom alleviation among pregnant women is not an "all or nothing" proposition.[6]

De Man et al. measured Disease Activity Scores (DAS) for 84 pregnant women with RA from before conception, when possible, to 26 weeks postpartum. There was an increase in the percent patients in remission from 17% in the first trimester to 27% in the third trimester, although the difference was not statistically significant. An analysis of disease activity scores over the course of pregnancy and postpartum demonstrated a mean pregnancy decrease and a mean postpartum increase.[5] Unlike the previous study, de Man et al. did not find any difference in disease activity between RF-positive and RF-negative women. There were also no differences among anti-cyclic citrullinated peptide (CCP)-positive and anti-CCP-negative women.[5]

Pathogenesis

The mechanism by which amelioration of RA symptoms occurs in pregnant women is not completely understood. Human leukocyte antigen (HLA) genes have been implicated in the pathogenesis of RA, and HLA alloantigens present in the fetus may provide an explanation for the change in immunologic response during pregnancy.[1] Nelson et al. analyzed maternal–fetal disparity in HLA alloantigens for 57 pregnancies of 41 women with RA. Seventy-six percent of women experiencing improvement or remission showed disparity in HLA-DRB1, DQA, and DQB, suggesting pregnancy-induced remission may result from a maternal immune response to paternal HLA antigens.[4]

Recently, attempts to explain the immunologic response during pregnancy have focused on the cytokine profiles of pregnant women with RA, a hypothesized shift in the T_H1 and T_H2 balance, and the role of regulatory T cells. Muñoz-Valle et al. studied the cytokine and hormone profiles of ten pregnant women with systemic lupus erythematosus (SLE), four pregnant women with RA, and 13 healthy pregnant controls from the first trimester through 1 month postpartum. When compared to SLE or normal controls, RA patients had a significantly increased level of interferon (IFN)-γ in the first trimester, decreasing in both trimesters and postpartum. Rheumatoid arthritis patients also experienced a significant increase in interleukin (IL)-10 mRNA expression level during the first trimester and a significant decrease in levels of IL-4 mRNA expression in all periods. Increased levels of matrix metalloproteinase (MMP)-9 activity were also observed in RA pregnant women.[7] These data, along with other study results, led the authors to conclude that the complex immune response involved in pregnancy cannot be described with an unambiguous cytokine profile.[7] Østensen et al. evaluated the changes in levels of circulating cytokines, focusing on the T_H1–T_H2 balance in a sample that included 19 pregnant women with RA, healthy pregnant controls, and nonpregnant women. During pregnancy, there was an increase of the inflammatory cytokines IL-1Ra and sTNFR. On the other hand, levels of IFN-γ and IL-10, both markers of a T_H1 and T_H2 response, were low or undetectable.[8] Förger et al. studied the association of disease activity and CD4+CD25$_{high}$ regulatory T cells in 12 pregnant women with RA and 14 healthy controls. In the majority of RA patients and in all healthy controls, the percentage of CD4+CD25$_{high}$ T cells was higher in the third trimester than during the postpartum period.[9] It remains for future researchers to weave these study findings into a coherent explanation of the mechanisms of RA amelioration and remission during pregnancy. A recent editorial, examining data (from a variety of sources) showing that an increased incidence of RA postpartum is accompanied by a reduced incidence during pregnancy, suggests that pregnancy merely postpones the clinical expression of the disease. Addressing the state of the immune system in these situations is consistent with the gene-environment model of RA pathogenesis.[10]

Management of Rheumatoid Arthritis During Pregnancy

It is unfortunate that well-designed and adequately powered studies of the safety profile of medications used to treat RA remain the exception rather than the rule.[11] Much of the information about the teratogenic effects of current RA treatment modalities is derived from small case studies, anecdotal evidence, animal models, or risk ratings from the U.S. Food and Drug Administration. Table 7.1 identifies the risk profile and current recommendations for the use of anti-inflammatories and DMARDs during pregnancy. The biologic agents deserve special mention, since it is estimated that up to 50% of RA patients will be using these drugs in the near future. No data is available to guide us when evaluating their use in pregnancy. Nevertheless, when large surveys of rheumatologists have been undertaken, anecdotal experiences from most rheumatologists indicate no increased risks for congenital malformations. Therefore, it is a matter of individual clinical judgment whether to continue these agents when pregnancy ensues, or to initiate them for active RA when a patient is considering becoming pregnant, or in the setting of a patient who has child-bearing potential with inadequate birth control.

Table 7.1 Recommendations for Use of Anti Inflammatory and Disease Modifying Antirheumatic Drugs during Pregnancy		
Treatment	Risk Profile	Recommendation
Anti-inflammatory agents		
Corticosteroids	Increase in oral clefts; dose-related intrauterine growth restriction.	May be used during pregnancy with minimal risk; lower doses will minimize risk.
Nonsteroidal anti-inflammatory drugs	Low risk for congenital malformations and miscarriage; significant risk after 32 weeks' gestation.	May be used during first trimester; discontinue use at or beyond 32 weeks' gestation.
Disease modifying antirheumatic drugs		
Methotrexate	Dose-related abnormalities of growth, craniofacies, limb development, and neurodevelopment.	Contraindicated in pregnancy; treatment should be discontinued at least 3 months prior to conception.

(continued)

45

Table 7.1 Continued

Treatment	Risk Profile	Recommendation
Sulfasalazine	Available data suggests low risk; no large well-controlled studies.	May be used during pregnancy; use should be accompanied by folic acid-containing vitamin supplements.
Leflunomide	Animal studies show increased risk for congenital malformations; minimal data in humans.	Contraindicated in pregnancy.
Hydroxychloroquine	Small studies show no increased risk for congenital malformations; not adequately studied in RA patients.	Teratogenic is unlikely; compatible with pregnancy.
Azathioprine	No increased risk for structural defects.	Compatible with pregnancy.
Cyclosporine	No increased risk for structural defects.	Compatible with pregnancy.
Chlorambucil	Insufficient data to determine teratogenic risk.	Contraindicated in pregnancy.
Cyclophosphamide	Risk for growth abnormalities, craniofacies, limb development, and neurodevelopment.	Contraindicated in pregnancy.
Biologics		
Etanercept	Insufficient data to determine teratogenic risk.	Physician discretion recommended.
Infliximab	Insufficient data to determine teratogenic risk.	Physician discretion recommended.
Adalimumab	Insufficient data to determine teratogenic risk.	Physician discretion recommended.
Golimumab	Insufficient data to determine teratogenic risk.	Physician discretion recommended.
Certolizumab pegol	Insufficient data to determine teratogenic risk.	Physician discretion recommended.
Rituximab	Insufficient data to determine teratogenic risk.	Physician discretion recommended.
Abatacept	Insufficient data to determine teratogenic risk.	Physician discretion recommended.
Anakinra	Insufficient data to determine teratogenic risk.	Physician discretion recommended.
Tocilizumab	Insufficient data to determine teratogenic risk.	Physician discretion recommended.

Adapted from Chambers 2006 and Østensen and Nelson 2004.

References

1. Østensen M, Nelson JL. Pregnancy. In St. Clair EM, Pisetsky DS, Haynes BF, eds., *Rheumatoid Arthritis*. Philadelphia: Lippincott Williams & Wilkins 2004:496–503.

2. Glyn J. The discovery and early use of cortisone. *J R Soc Med* 1998; 91(10):513–517.

3. Hench PS. The ameliorating effect of pregnancy on chronic atrophic (infectious rheumatoid) arthritis, fibrosis, and intermittent hydrarthrosis. *Proc Staff Meet Mayo Clin* 1938;13:161–167.

4. Nelson JL, Hughes KA, Smith AG, et al. Maternal-fetal disparity in HLA class II alloantigens and the pregnancy-induced amelioration of rheumatoid arthritis. *N Engl J Med* 1993;329(7):466–471.

5. de Man YA, Dolhain RJ, van de Geijn FE, et al. Disease activity of rheumatoid arthritis during pregnancy: Results from a nationwide prospective study. *Arthritis Rheum* 2008;59(9):1241–1248.

6. Barrett JH, Brennan P, Fiddler M, Silman AJ. Does rheumatoid arthritis remit during pregnancy and relapse postpartum? *Arthritis Rheum* 1999;42(6):1219–1227.

7. Muñoz-Valle JF, Vázquez-del Mercado M, Garc´a-Iglesias T, et al. T_H1/T_H2 cytokine profile, metalloprotease-9 activity and hormonal status in pregnant rheumatoid arthritis and systemic lupus erythematosus patients. *Clin Exp Immunol* 2003;131(2):377–384.

8. Østensen M, Förger F, Nelson JL, et al. Pregnancy in patients with rheumatic disease: Anti-inflammatory cytokines increase in pregnancy and decrease post partum. *Ann Rheum Dis* 2005;64(6):839–844.

9. Förger F, Marcoli N, Gadola S, et al. Pregnancy induces numerical and functional changes of CD4+CD25^{high} regulatory T cells in patients with rheumatoid arthritis. *Ann Rheum Dis* 2008;67(7):984–990.

10. Dolhain, Radboud J E M "Rheumatoid arthritis and pregnancy; not only for rheumatologists interested in female health issues. *Ann Rheum Dis* February 2010 Vol 69 pages 317–318

11. Chambers CD, Tutuncu ZN, Johnson D, Jones KL. Human pregnancy safety for agents used to treat rheumatoid arthritis: Adequacy of available information and strategies for developing post-marketing data. *Arthritis Res Ther* 2006;8(4):215.

Chapter 8

Outcome Measurement

Given the progressive systemic inflammatory nature of the disease, patients with rheumatoid arthritis (RA) may experience serious physical, mental, and social consequences resulting in a compromised quality of life. Decrements in physical function may be accompanied by diminished labor force participation and ability to perform activities of daily living, culminating in both direct and indirect costs to the patient and society.

The pioneering work of Drs. Robert Kaplan and J.W. Bush led health services researchers to recognize the importance of measuring patient well-being.[1] It is especially imperative that physicians measure the function and health status of their patients with RA at each visit. Studies have demonstrated that health assessment data obtained from questionnaires may be just as valuable as laboratory or imaging data in determining patient care,[2] identifying patients with work disability limitations,[2] and predicting mortality.[3] The administration of an arthritis health status questionnaire may seem an added burden to the busy practitioner. However, Pincus and Wolfe note that "simple clinical patient questionnaires save time and make us better physicians".[3]

Although there is no "gold standard" for assessing patient status in RA, numerous health status assessments have been developed to measure disease activity and functional ability in RA patients. Although the majority of these instruments are used primarily in clinical trials, the Multidimensional Health Assessment Questionnaire (MDHAQ), the CLINHAQ, and the Clinical Disease Activity Index (CDAI), discussed here, may be easily incorporated into busy clinical practices.

American College of Rheumatology Core Set of Disease Activity Measures

The American College of Rheumatology (ACR) core set of disease activity measures were developed for a specified purpose; they originate from clinical trials, and they were developed to discriminate between a response to a therapeutic agent and a response to a placebo. This core set is one of several RA pooled indices and is comprised of seven items selected on the basis of ability to measure improvement in RA symptoms, sensitivity to change, and potential to predict long-term outcome.[4] The ACR core set includes tender joint count, swollen joint count, patient's assessment of pain, patient's global assessment of disease activity, physician's global assessment of disease activity, patient's assessment of physical function, and an acute-phase reactant value, either erythrocyte sedimentation rate (ESR) or C-reactive protein.[4] The initial tender and swollen joint count recommended by ACR included an assessment of 68 and 66 joints, respectively. At present, the most frequently used measure is a tender and swollen 28-joint count that includes shoulder, elbow, wrist, the first through fifth metacarpophalangeal, and the first through fifth proximal inter-phalangeal.[5] An assessment of feet and ankle joints is excluded due to potential confounding with other conditions.[6] The patient's assessment of pain, patient's global assessment of disease activity, and the physician's global assessment of disease activity may be measured on a visual analog scale of 10 cm or a Likert scale assessing current level of pain or disease activity. Instruments used to measure the patient's assessment of physical function include the Arthritis Impact Measurement Scales (AIMS), Health Assessment Questionnaire (HAQ), and the McMaster Toronto Arthritis Patient Preference Disability Questionnaire (MACTAR).[4]

Disease Activity Score

The Disease Activity Score (DAS), initially developed in 1990, is another pooled index of RA disease activity. The origin of the DAS is more relevant to the practice of medicine when compared to the ACR measures; this is because the instrument was developed from an observational cohort of patients in routine clinical practice. The components of the original DAS include the Ritchie articular index, a 44 swollen joint count, ESR, and a general health assessment measured on a 10 cm visual analog scale.[7] The DAS is scored using a complex formula that includes the square root of the Ritchie articular index and the natural log of the ESR.[6] In part due to this complex scoring formula, the DAS was subsequently modified.[6] The modified DAS, referred to as the DAS28, replaces the Ritchie articular index and the 44 swollen joint count with a 28-joint count.[8] Other derivations of the DAS include the Simplified Disease Activity Index (SDAI) and the Clinical Disease Activity Index (CDAI). The SDAI and the CDAI both include a 28 swollen joint count, 28 tender joint count, patient global assessment, and physician global assessment. The SDAI includes a C-reactive protein measure that is excluded from the CDAI.[6] Both the SDAI and CDAI are scored as a simple additive function, making either index convenient for use in a clinical setting.

Measures of Physical Function and Quality of Life

Although current treatments may moderate the course of the disease, patients with RA may experience physical limitations ranging from mild to severe over the course of their lifetime. Functional and quality-of-life limitations experienced by RA patients can be assessed using either disease-specific or generic measures. Disease-specific instruments are designed to measure those aspects of a disease most likely to respond to therapy and are specific to individual conditions, such as arthritis or heart disease.[9] Generic instruments measure the overall health and well-being of the individual.

The most commonly used disease-specific RA instruments to measure physical function are the HAQ, the Multidimensional Health Assessment

Questionnaire (MDHAQ), AIMS, and MACTAR. The HAQ Disability Index (included in Appendix 2) contains 20 questions that ask respondents to report the degree of difficulty performing activities in eight categories: dressing and grooming, arising, eating, walking, hygiene, reach, grip, and errands and chores. Responses are scored on a 4-point scale of difficulty: no difficulty, some difficulty, much difficulty, unable to do. The questionnaire also asks respondents to report whether any aids or devices are used for their activities and whether help is required from another person in performing selected tasks.[10] The HAQ Disability Index score ranges from 0 to 3, with increments of 0.125. Scores of <1.0 indicate mild limitations, scores of 1.0–2.0 indicate moderate limitations, and scores >2.0 indicate severe limitations. Use of aids or devices or assistance from others in performing selected tasks may be incorporated into the final score.[10]

Due to the way activities are grouped within each of the eight HAQ categories, a patient may improve in several activities but show no change in HAQ scores.[11] This, along with other limitations of the HAQ, led to the development of the MDHAQ. The MDHAQ is a two-page questionnaire that was designed to be easily administered in the physician's office to assess functional capacity and disease activity. The MDHAQ measures physical function in ten activities, pain, global status, fatigue, self-report joint count, review of systems, recent medical events, morning stiffness, and change of status.[12] Scoring templates are included with the questionnaire and may be scored in less than 15 seconds.[11] Equally effective for administration and scoring by busy physicians is the CLINHAQ.[2] The CLINQHAQ, which has been administered by Wolfe and Pincus in excess of 100,000 times to 25,000 patients in their clinical practice,[2] includes the HAQ disability scale, global assessments of pain, fatigue, sleep disturbance, and severity, and assessments of health status.[2]

The AIMS was originally introduced in 1980[13] and subsequently revised as the AIMS2 in 1992.[14] The AIMS2 consists of 57 core items categorized into 12 dimensions: mobility level, walking and bending, hand and finger function, arm function, self-care, household tasks, arthritis pain, work, social activities, support from family and friends, tension, and mood. Its use in clinical practice is limited due to the length of the questionnaire, which may take from 20 to 30 minutes to complete. A short form of the AIMS2, the AIMS2-SF was developed and validated in 1997. While retaining the psychometric properties of the AIMS2, the AIMS2-SF consists of 26 items and is easily administered in a clinical practice setting.[15]

The MACTAR differs from the HAQ and AIMS in that it allows patients to target specific functional tasks for improvement. In addition to enumerating functional areas for improvement, the patient is asked about limitations relative to activities around the house, activities at work, athletic and nonathletic activities, and social activities. Patients are also queried about their ability to perform an array of tasks without the use of splints or mechanical aids.[16] Because it uses patient nomination of areas for functional improvement, the MACTAR may be sensitive as a measure of physical change.[10]

The most widely used generic quality-of-life measure is the Short Form 36 (SF-36). The SF-36 measures eight dimensions of health status: physical functioning, role limitations, bodily pain, social functioning, general mental health, social role limitations, vitality, and general health perceptions.[17] Two summary scores are derived from these eight dimensions: the physical component summary (PCS) and the mental component summary (MSC).[17] In clinical trials testing the effectiveness of RA treatments, the SF-36 is an excellent complement to the HAQ, AIMS, or MACTAR because it includes a measure of emotional well-being not present in the former instruments.

There are very few RA disease-specific quality-of-life measures. Whalley et al. developed the RAQOL,[18] a 30-item instrument that includes measures of self-care, indoor and outdoor activities, emotions and conditions, and interpersonal relations. The RAQOL has demonstrated excellent psychometric properties including test-retest reliability > 0.9 and an ability to discriminate between groups with different levels of disease activity and severity.[19]

While the disease remains active, monthly visits to a rheumatologist are recommended to successfully monitor patient progress and identify any necessary changes to the patient's treatment regimen

The recommendation that patients with RA visit the rheumatologist once a month comes from a very influential trial published in 2004, called TICORA,[20] in which the investigators compared patient outcomes from two strategies involving nonbiologic disease-modifying antirheumatic drugs (DMARDs). Patients were randomly assigned to an intensive outpatient regimen (in which patients were seen every month by the same rheumatologist and their disease activity score was calculated) or to routine rheumatologic care. The clear-cut winning strategy was a rigorous monthly regimen in which intensive administration of nonbiologic DMARDs (and aggressive corticosteroid management) were applied to achieve and maintain a predefined low disease activity score (DAS ≤ 2.4). Follow-up of this study in later publications indicated that the benefit (both clinical and radiologic) was maintained for an additional 5 years. Although outpatient and drug administration costs were higher in the intensive treatment arm, the investigators point out that this was offset by higher inpatient costs in the routine group; the total community costs were equal for both regimens as a result. This study points out that it is not necessarily the drug per se that makes the difference (although some argue this point) but the intensity of the regimen and the timing of the aggressive approach (in the early years of RA) that are most important.

References

1. Kaplan RM, Bush JW, Berry CC. Health status: types of validity and the index of well-being. *Health Serv Res* 1976;11(4):478–507.

2. Wolfe F, Pincus T. Listening to the patient: A practical guide to self-report questionnaires in clinical care. *Arthritis Rheum* 1999;42(9):1797–1808.

3. Pincus T, Wolfe F. Patient questionnaires for clinical research and improved standard patient care: Is it better to have 80% of the information in 100% of patients or 100% of the information in 5% of patients? *J Rheumatol* 2005;32(4):575–577.

4. Felson DT, Anderson JJ, Boers M, et al. The American College of Rheumatology preliminary core set of disease activity measures for rheumatoid arthritis clinical trials. *Arthritis Rheum* 1993;36(6):729–740.

5. Fuchs HA, Brooks RH, Callahan LF, Pincus T. A simplified twenty-eight joint quantitative articular index in rheumatoid arthritis. *Arthritis Rheum* 1989; 32(5):531–537.

6. Aletaha D, Smolen JS. Outcome measurement in rheumatoid arthritis: Disease activity. In Hochberg MC et al., eds., *Rheumatoid Arthritis*, 1st edition. Philadelphia: Mosby 2009:225–230.

7. van der Heijde DM, van'tHof MA, van Riel PL, et al. Judging disease activity in clinical practice in rheumatoid arthritis: First step in the development of a disease activity score. *Ann Rheum Dis* 1990;49(11):916–920.

8. Prevoo ML, van't Hof MA, Kuper HH, et al. Modified disease activity scores that include twenty-eight joint counts. *Arthritis Rheum* 1995;38(1):44–48.

9. Tugwell P, Idzerda L, Wells GA. Generic quality-of-life assessment in rheumatoid arthritis. *Am J Manag Care* 2007;13(Suppl 9):S224-S236.

10. Ward MM. Physical function. In Hochberg MC et al., eds., *Rheumatoid Arthritis*, 1st edition. Philadelphia: Mosby 2009:231–236.

11. Pincus T, Yazici Y, Bergman M. Development of a multi-dimensional health assessment questionnaire (MDHAQ) for the infrastructure of standard clinical care. *Clin Exp Rheumatol* 2005;23(5 Suppl 39):S19-S28.

12. http://mdhaq.org/Default.aspx.

13. Meenan RF, Gertman PM, Mason JH, Dunaif R. The Arthritis Impact Measurement Scales. Further investigations of a health status measure. *Arthritis Rheum* 1982;25(9):1048–1053.

14. Meenan RF, Mason JH, Anderson JJ, et al. AIMS2. The content and properties of a revised and expanded Arthritis Impact Measurement Scales health status questionnaire. *Arthritis Rheum* 1992;35(1):1–10.

15. Guillemin F, Coste J, Pouchot J, et al. The AIMS2-SF: A short form of the Arthritis Impact Measurement Scales 2. French Quality of Life in Rheumatology Group. *Arthritis Rheum* 1997;40(7):1267–1274.

16. Tugwell P, Bombardier C, Buchanan WW, et al. The MACTAR patient preference disability questionnaire: An individualized functional priority approach for assessing improvements in physical disability in clinical trials in rheumatoid arthritis. *J Rheumatol* 1987;14(3):446–451.

17. Ware JE, Sherbourne CD. The MOS 36-item short-form health survey (SF-36). I. Conceptual framework and item selection. *Med Care* 1992;30(6):473–483.

18. Whalley D, McKenna SP, De Jong Z, van der Heijde D. Quality of life in rheumatoid arthritis. *Br J Rheumatol* 1997;36(8):884–888.

19. de Jong Z, van der Heijde D, McKenna SP, Whalley D. The reliability and construct validity of the RAQoL: A rheumatoid arthritis-specific quality of life instrument. *Br J Rheumatol* 1997;36(8):878–882.

20. Grigor C, Capell H, Stirling A et al. Effect of a treatment strategy of tight control for rheumatoid arthritis (the TICORA study): A single-blind randomized controlled trial. *Lancet* 2004;364(9430):263–269.

Chapter 9

Laboratory and Imaging Assessments

The primary tools at the clinician's disposal for the detection and assessment of rheumatoid arthritis (RA) and its attendant damage are laboratory tests, radiographic examination (x-rays), ultrasonography (US), magnetic resonance imaging (MRI) and, although rarely used in clinical practice,[1] computed tomography (CT). Laboratory tests are used to determine the presence of autoantibodies for rheumatoid factor (RF) and anti-cyclic citrullinated peptide (CCP). Radiographic examination is readily available to clinicians and is the most frequently used method to determine joint damage and response to therapeutic intervention. Ultrasound allows the detection of early inflammatory soft-tissue lesions and early erosive bone lesions,[2] whereas MRI and CT offer the advantage of a pictorial view of joint damage (and in the case of MRI, inflammation) from a multidimensional perspective. The strengths and limitations of these assessments are discussed below.

Rheumatoid Factor and Anti-Cyclic Citrullinated Peptide

Both RF and anti-CCP antibodies have been shown to predate the onset of RA.[3,4] Traditionally, the antibody test for RF has been used as a diagnostic marker for RA. However, although RF is present in approximately 80% of RA patients,[5] its use as a diagnostic marker for RA is limited because of both sensitivity and specificity issues: RF may also be present in both healthy individuals[5] and in individuals with other autoimmune and infectious diseases.[6] Of the rheumatoid factors, some investigations have revealed that IgA-RF demonstrates the highest sensitivity prior to disease onset, whereas IgM-RF has the highest sensitivity subsequent to disease onset.[3]

The anti-CCP antibody test, recently introduced as a diagnostic and prognostic tool,[7] determines the presence of the anti-CCP resulting from antibodies to modified (citrullinated) arginine residues.[7] The utility of the anti-CCP antibody test is twofold. First, it is diagnostically useful as a marker for identifying RA in patients with early undifferentiated arthritis and a negative RF.[8] Second, anti-CCP antibodies have prognostic utility with respect to radiographic outcomes.[6,7] Kroot et al. reported that anti-CCP-positive patients developed significantly more severe radiologic damage after 6 years of follow-up than did anti-CCP-negative patients.[5] Despite these advantages, it is important to note that between 33% and 40% of RA patients do not have anti-CCP or RF antibodies.[8]

Avouac et al. conducted a systematic review of the literature to determine the sensitivity (i.e., the proportion of people with RA who have a positive test result) and specificity (i.e., the proportion of people without RA who have a negative test result) of RF as well as two generations of anti-CCP antibody tests (anti-CCP1 and anti-CCP2).[9] Within a population of RA patients, the mean sensitivity and specificity of RF were 60% and 79%, respectively.[9] The mean sensitivity of the anti-CCP1 test among RA patients was 53%, whereas the corresponding sensitivity for the anti-CCP2 was 58%.[9] The mean specificity for the anti-CCP1 and anti-CCP2 among RA patients was 96% and 95%, respectively.[9] Additional analysis indicated that, compared to RF, anti-CCP antibodies appear to be better predictors of the development of RA among patients with early undifferentiated arthritis. The odds ratio of developing RA was 20 (95% CI 14–31) for anti-CCP1 and 25 (95% CI 18–35) for anti-CCP2.[9] A meta-analysis by Nishimura et al. reached similar conclusions with regard to the sensitivity and specificity of RF and anti-CCP antibodies.[6] An analysis of anti-CCP antibodies in the presence of the shared epitope (SE), indicated that the presence of the SE enhances the predictive value of anti-CCP antibodies in predicting the risk of future development of RA.[4] In general, anti-CCP antibody testing augments RF testing for both diagnostic and therapeutic purposes; together, they increase our overall diagnostic ability (CCP may be positive when RF is negative) and prognosis (CCP does appear to mark patients with a worse prognosis).

Radiography

Radiography is the most common method for establishing the presence of structural damage in RA and determining therapeutic response. Radiographs reflect the structural damage that results from cumulative disease activity[10] and serve as surrogate indicators of functional capacity and work disability.[10] A number of scoring methods are used to rate the presence and severity of structural damage. These methods, which include Larson Score, Scott Modification of Larsen's Method, Ratingen Score, Sharp's Method, Genant's Modification of Sharp's Method, and van der Heijde's Modification of Sharp's Method, are primarily used in clinical trials.[10] What they share in common is a scoring system for joint erosion and/or joint space narrowing. The Simple Erosion Narrowing Score (SENS) is a simple count of the number of eroded and narrowed joints[10] and is recommended for clinicians interested in reading and scoring the radiographs of their RA patients.

In its favor, radiography offers a readily available, low cost assessment of cumulative joint damage[11] that produces very few false positives.[8] With most facilities now using digital techniques with much better resolution, its diagnostic sensitivity and specificity have substantially improved. Radiography may also aid in differentiating RA from other joint conditions, including psoriatic arthritis, osteoarthritis, gouty arthritis, and neoplasms.[11] The disadvantages of radiography include its two-dimensional representation of a three-dimensional pathology,[10,11] lack of sensitivity in detecting the presence of early disease,[11,12] inability to assess synovitis and other soft-tissue changes,[1] and poor sensitivity in detecting bone erosions.[12]

Ultrasonography

The application of US in the assessment of RA represents a significant diagnostic advancement because of its ability to detect early inflammatory soft-tissue lesions and early erosive bone lesions.[2] In particular, US is able to detect the presence of fluid in joints, bursae, and tendon sheaths, as well as inflammation at the enthesitis of tendons and ligaments.[11] Clinicians are just beginning to use this technique to guide injections and aspirations, and the future use of US in this area appears promising. The detection of early inflammation is made possible by the use of color and power Doppler US, enabling the clinician to distinguish between active and inactive joint processes.[2] Although US has several advantages relative to radiography and MRI, including its ability to visualize a three-dimensional plane and scan numerous joints in a short period of time,[13] it is operator-dependent and there remain issues regarding its reproducibility, validity, and responsiveness to change.[13] Factors affecting the reliability of US findings include interobserver reliability, intraobserver reliability, and intermachine reliability.[13] Only a handful of studies have analyzed the reliability of US findings relative to other imaging methods,[13] and there is no data on the correlation between US findings and later radiographic or functional status.[14] Most significantly, perhaps, the use of US to monitor disease progression in RA is limited by a lack of consensus as to the specific number and localization of joints that require examination.[1]

Szkudlarek et al. studied the sensitivity, specificity, and accuracy of US relative to MRI, conventional radiography, and clinical examination in the metatarsophalangeal (MTP) joints of RA patients.[15] The results of their study indicate that, compared with MRI, US was more sensitive and accurate than conventional radiography and clinical examination in the detection of destructive and inflammatory changes in the MTP joints of patients with RA.[15] In a separate investigation, Szkudlarek et al. assessed the sensitivity, specificity, and accuracy of US in detecting signs of inflammation and destruction in the second to fifth metacarpophalangeal (MCP) joints.[16] Similar to their findings about the effectiveness of US in the evaluation of MTP joints, relative to MRI, US demonstrated a greater sensitivity than radiography in detecting bone erosions and had equal specificity.[16] In one of the only long-term follow-up studies comparing radiography, US, and MRI for the detection of bone erosions and synovitis in the finger joints of RA patients, Scheel et al. demonstrated that US was more sensitive than MRI for the detection of very small fluid accumulations in the proximal interphalangeal (PIP) joints.[14]

Magnetic Resonance Imaging

There are those who suggest that MRI is the most sensitive imaging modality currently available. [17-19] Unlike radiography or US, MRI is able to provide visualization of the joints in three orthogonal planes.[20] It also offers the advantage of avoiding ionizing radiation while providing excellent detail of the bone and surrounding soft tissue, as well as possessing increased sensitivity for erosion detection.[20] In particular, MRI enables an assessment of the synovial membrane, intra- and extra-articular fluid collections, cartilage, bone, ligaments, tendons, and tendon sheaths.[11] The disadvantages of MRI include its cost and availability[20] and that evaluation is limited to a specific field of view and a few joints per session.[11] Further, the advancement of a low-field office-based MRI for clinical purposes has yet to be validated, and a recent report by the American College of Rheumatology[21] urges caution in the widespread adoption of this technique for diagnostic and therapeutic decision making.

Careful consideration is advised before embracing MRI as the panacea for the detection of erosive disease in RA patients. Although MRI may be more sensitive than radiography in identifying erosions early in the disease process,[21] Goldbach-Mansky et al. call for caution, citing the difficulty of interpreting early MRI lesions and noting, for example, that after 2 years, only one of four erosions detected by MRI went on to become documented radiographic erosions.[22] On the other hand, after reviewing studies with follow-up periods of 1, 2, 6, and 10 years, Østergaard et al. conclude that MRI is a highly significant predictor of radiographic erosions.[1] Recent studies do support the fact that bone lesions (including "bone edema") detected by MRI do, in fact, have a physiologic basis in rheumatoid inflammation,[23] but whether they will go on to mark actual bone destruction is not yet known. A very recent study[24] and accompanying editorial[25] point out that MRI bone lesions have a very poor positive predictive value for true bone erosions on x-ray (many are entirely reversible over time) but their negative predictive value (x-ray erosions appear not to develop in the absence of bone lesions) is very strong. Therefore, what we know at present is that MRI provides an extremely sensitive tool to detect RA inflammation in soft tissues (synovium, tendon sheaths, entheses, etc.), as well as in bone. This is most useful diagnostically, but the employment of this information for specific treatment decisions (for example, whether or not to use a tumor necrosis factor [TNF] agent) remains to be determined.

Computed Tomography

Computed tomography provides a three-dimensional visualization of joints and other structures using a multiplanar reconstruction of x-ray imaging that enables the visualization of calcified tissue with high resolution.[1] This powerful imaging modality makes CT the standard reference for locating and evaluating destruction of calcified tissue.[1] Although powerful, CT does not adequately visualize soft-tissue changes of articular structures.[1] As noted earlier, CT is rarely used in routine rheumatologic clinical practice related to the joint disease of RA, since MRI has largely substituted CT for soft-tissue imaging. Given the requirement for additional ionizing radiation required by the CT techniques, the use of CT is currently relegated to very specific instances in which three-dimensional imaging is a necessity for diagnostic and therapeutic decision making.

References

1. Østergaard M, Pedersen SJ, Døhn UM. Imaging in rheumatoid arthritis: Status and recent advances for magnetic resonance imaging, ultrasonography, computed tomography and conventional radiography. *Best Pract Res Clin Rheumatol* 2008;22(6):1019–1044.

2. Backhaus M. Sonography. In Hochberg MC et al., eds., *Rheumatoid Arthritis*, 1st edition. Philadelphia: Mosby 2009:267–274.

3. Rantapää-Dahlqvist S. What happens before the onset of rheumatoid arthritis? *Curr Opin Rheumatol* 2009;21(3):272–278.

4. Berglin E, Padyukov L, Sundin U, et al. A combination of autoantibodies to cyclic citrullinated peptide (CCP) and HLA-DRB1 locus antigens is strongly associated with future onset of rheumatoid arthritis. *Arthritis Res Ther* 2004;6(4):R303–308.

5. Kroot EJ, de Jong BA, van Leeuwen MA, et al. The prognostic value of anti-cyclic citrullinated peptide antibody in patients with recent-onset rheumatoid arthritis. *Arthritis Rheum* 2000;43(8):1831–1835.

6. Nishimura K, Sugiyama D, Kogata Y, et al. Meta-analysis: Diagnostic accuracy of anti-cyclic citrullinated peptide antibody and rheumatoid factor for rheumatoid arthritis. *Ann Intern Med* 2007;146(11):797–808.

7. Quinn MA, Gough AK, Green MJ, et al. Anti-CCP antibodies measured at disease onset help identify seronegative rheumatoid arthritis and predict radiological and functional outcome. *Rheumatology* 2005;45(4):478–480.

8. Pincus T. Advantages and limitations of quantitative measures to assess rheumatoid arthritis: joint counts, radiographs, laboratory tests, and patient. *Bull NYU Hosp Joint Dis* 2006;64(1–2):32–39.

9. Avouac J, Gossec L, Dougados M. Diagnostic and predictive value of anti-cyclic citrullinated protein antibodies in rheumatoid arthritis: A systematic literature review. *Ann Rheum Dis* 2006;65(7):845–851.

10. van der Heijde D. Radiography. In Hochberg MC et al., eds., *Rheumatoid Arthritis*, 1st edition. Philadelphia: Mosby 2009:260–266.

11. Østergaard M, Ejbjerg B, Szkudlarek M. Imaging in early rheumatoid arthritis: Roles of magnetic resonance imaging, ultrasonography, conventional radiography and computed tomography. *Best Pract Res Clin Rheumatol* 2005;19(1):91–116.

12. Døhn UM, Ejbjerg BJ, Court-Payen M, et al. Are bone erosions detected by magnetic resonance imaging and ultrasonography true erosions? A comparison with computed tomography in rheumatoid arthritis metacarpophalangeal joints. *Arthritis Res Ther* 2006;8(4):R110.

13. Wakefield RJ, Balint P, Szkudlarek M, et al. for the OMERACT 7 Special Interest Group. Musculoskeletal ultrasound including definitions for ultrasonographic pathology. *J Rheumatol* 2005;32(12):2485–2487.

14. Scheel AK, Hermann KG, Ohrndorf S, et al. Prospective 7-year follow-up imaging study comparing radiography, ultrasonography, and magnetic resonance imaging in rheumatoid arthritis finger joints. *Ann Rheum Dis* 2006;65(5):595–600.

15. Szkudlarek M, Narvestad E, Klarlund M, et al. Ultrasonography of the metatarsophalangeal joints in rheumatoid arthritis: Comparison with magnetic resonance imaging, conventional radiography, and clinical examination. *Arthritis Rheum* 2004;50(7):2103–2112.

16. Szkudlarek M, Klarlund M, Narvestad E, et al. Ultrasonography of the metacarpophalangeal and proximal interphalangeal joints in rheumatoid arthritis: A

comparison with magnetic resonance imaging, conventional radiography, and clinical examination. *Arthritis Res Ther* 2006;8(2):R52.

17. Sugimoto H, Takeda A, Masuyama J, et al. Early-stage rheumatoid arthritis: Diagnostic accuracy of MR imaging. *Radiology* 1996;198(1):185–192.

18. Østergaard M, Hansen M., Stoltenberg M, et al. New radiographic bone erosions in the wrists of patients with rheumatoid arthritis are detectable with magnetic resonance imaging a median of two years earlier. *Arthritis Rheum* 2003;48(8):2128–2131.

19. Klarlund M, Østergaard M, Jensen KE, et al. Magnetic resonance imaging, radiography, and scintigraphy of the finger joints: One-year follow-up of patients with early arthritis. The TIRA Group. *Rheum Dis* 2000;59(7):521–528.

20. Freeston JE, Conaghan PG. Outcome measurement in rheumatoid arthritis: Magnetic resonance imaging. In Hochberg MC et al., eds., *Rheumatoid Arthritis*, 1st edition. Philadelphia: Mosby 2009:275–278.

21. American College of Rheumatology. Extremity Magnetic Resonance Imaging Task Force. Extremity magnetic resonance imaging in rheumatoid arthritis: Report of the American College of Rheumatology Extremity Magnetic Resonance Imaging Task Force. *Arthritis Rheum* 2006; 54(4):1034–1047.

22. Goldbach-Mansky R, Woodburn J, Yao L, Lipsky PE. Magnetic resonance imaging in the evaluation of bone damage in rheumatoid arthritis: A more precise image or just a more expensive one? *Arthritis Rheum* 2003;48(3):585–589.

23. Jimenez-Boj E, Nobauer-Huhmann I, Hanslik-Schnabel B et al. Bone erosions and bone marrow edema as defined by magnetic resonance imaging reflect true bone marrow inflammation in rheumatoid arthritis. *Arthritis Rheum* 2007;56(4):1118–1124.

24. Mundwiler ML, Maranian P, Brown DH, et al. The utility of MRI in predicting radiographic erosions in the metatarsophalangeal joints of the rheumatoid foot: A prospective longitudinal cohort study. *Arthritis Res Ther* 2009;11(3):R94.

25. McQueen FM, Dalbeth N. Predicting joint damage in rheumatoid arthritis using MRI scanning. *Arthritis Res Ther* 2009;11(5):124.

Chapter 10

Differential Diagnosis

As might be inferred from the previous chapters, no single test is available to the clinician to confirm a diagnosis of rheumatoid arthritis (RA). Rather, the diagnosis of RA must be made using the composite findings from clinical examination, laboratory assessments, radiographic examination, and perhaps sonography or magnetic resonance imaging (MRI). The convergence of these diagnostic tools is explicitly acknowledged in the American College of Rheumatology's 1987 Classification Criteria of Acute Arthritis of Rheumatoid Arthritis (see Chapter 2) that requires the presence of at least four of seven of the following criteria: morning stiffness, arthritis of three or more joint areas, arthritis of hand joints, symmetric arthritis, rheumatoid nodules, serum rheumatoid factor, and radiographic changes.[1] However, it is important to note that these are "classification" criteria and not diagnostic criteria. By definition, classification criteria are highly specific because they are used for research purposes—so that all investigators can agree on the diagnosis—and to avoid misclassification. This is important, for example, when doing genetic studies. Nevertheless, we see patients in their early stages well before they develop all of the "full-blown" signs and symptoms of RA or before they evolve into having met classification criteria. How do we make a diagnosis then? What about the patient who presents with just a week or two of arthritis in a couple of joints? Is that patient's arthritis going to evolve into RA? Does the patient have another acute illness (such as an infection, or gout)? Or is the patient's condition going to go away by the end of the month? This challenge is addressed here.

The examination of a patient presenting with an acute or chronic polyarthritis should begin with a complete history and review of symptoms, including an assessment of articular, periarticular, and extra-articular manifestations (refer to Chapter 5 for RA-specific signs and symptoms). The clinician should determine whether the patient has had any previous episodes or previous serious infections, including fungal infections, viral infections, exposures outside of the United States, tuberculosis, and hepatitis B or C.[2] Laboratory and imaging assessments should be completed concurrently with the physical examination. Patients with early arthritis whose disease may progress to RA generally have higher levels of acute-phase parameters such as C-reactive protein (CRP) or erythrocyte sedimentation rate (ESR).[3] Conversely, some patients who present with acute polyarthritis and a normal ESR and CRP will turn out to have a viral infection, such as hepatitis B or C (personal observations of the author).

In general, one can separate the differential diagnostic possibilities into two groups—one for acute monoarticular and one for acute polyarticular arthritis, recognizing that this is only an approximation and not an iron-clad rule. For patients who present with a single swollen joint, the most serious issue for the clinician is to make sure that this is not an infectious or a crystal-induced arthritis. The two situations require dramatically different treatment approaches. In either case, aspiration of the joint for synovial fluid analysis (including culture and sensitivity, crystal analysis) is essential. In some situations (for example, when the patient has already been given antibiotics), the patient may need to be treated as if he or she had a septic joint until circumstances evolve that prove otherwise. In other scenarios, a patient with crystal-proven calcium pyrophosphate dihydrate deposition (CPPD) disease (pseudogout attack) may have a concomitant septic joint—thus, the culture should be done, and an open mind to this possibility must be maintained.

Many patients who present to the primary care physician with an acute or short-duration inflammatory polyarthritis do not become chronically ill or go on to develop RA. However, the longer they have the polyarthritis at presentation, the greater the possibility that it will become chronic. In general, if the patient has had signs and symptoms for <6 weeks, the possibilities include acute viral and bacterial infections. The differential diagnosis here includes acute viral infections (rubella, parvovirus, hepatitis B or C, human immunodeficiency virus [HIV] disease) and rarely bacterial endocarditis or acute rheumatic fever.

For patients with longer-duration polyarthritis, defined here as a condition or disease persisting >6 weeks, any number of disorders should be differentiated from RA, including chronic crystalline arthropathy, infectious arthritis with tuberculosis (TB) or fungi, spondyloarthropathies or reactive arthritis, arthritis related to connective tissue diseases or systemic vasculitis, Behçet's disease, adult Still's disease, palindromic rheumatism, sarcoidosis, polymyalgia rheumatica, remitting seronegative synovitis with pitting edema, malignancy-related arthritis, hypertrophic osteoarthropathy, osteoarthritis, fibromyalgia, infiltrative disorders, hemochromatosis, endocrinopathies, hemophilic arthropathy, and pigmented villonodular synovitis.[2]

Significant findings from the physical examination should be used to determine the diagnosis of RA in the patient with a chronic polyarthritis. In so doing, the following five rules can be used as guidelines in establishing the differential diagnosis of patients with chronic polyarthritis.[4]

1. Knowledge of the pathogenesis of the disease is of critical importance to predict physical findings.
2. The distribution of joint involvement around the body provides important clues to the differential diagnosis.
3. The unique involvement of the hand and foot (i.e., which joints or groups of joints are involved) refines the differential diagnosis into more specific diseases.
4. Extra-articular manifestations observed in the individual diseases often supply insight toward the diagnosis.
5. Certain conditions produce symptoms out of proportion to physical findings; awareness of this fact facilitates differential diagnosis.

The application of these rules to a determination of a diagnosis of RA is outlined here.

Rule 1: Pathogenetic aspects predict physical findings. Because the synovium is the primary pathogenetic focus of the disease, clinical evidence for the presence of RA is manifest in an inflammatory response in the synovium resulting in

enlarged, warm, and tender joints that exude copious amounts of inflammatory fluid.[3] An MRI can be used to document this feature if there is doubt.
The author has sometimes used bone radionuclide scintigraphy for the same
purpose, to "rule out" inflammation if the physical exam is equivocal or the
patient is especially obese.

*Rule 2: Distribution of joint involvement around the body provides clues to the diag-
nosis.* The distribution of joint involvement in RA is bilateral and symmetric.
Large, as well as small joints may be affected, and joint involvement appears
in both the upper and lower extremities.[3] This pattern is very common in
established disease. In early-onset RA, however, there may be fewer joints
involved and the overall distribution may not have evolved completely into a
fully bilateral and symmetric pattern.

Rule 3: Distribution in the hand and foot refines the specific of the diagnosis.
Rheumatoid arthritis almost always involves the metacarpophalangeal (MCP)
joints and the wrist, in addition to the interphalangeal (IP) joints. It is criti-
cally important for a proper differential diagnosis to distinguish, on physical
examination, between RA involvement of the wrist and OA affecting the first
carpometacarpal (CMC) joint.[3] In the foot, the metatarsophalangeal (MTP)
joints are involved in the earliest stages, and sometimes grasping the fifth
MTP joint or squeezing across all of the MTP joints will produce pain and
show swelling.

Rule 4: Extra-articular features supply additional insight into the diagnosis. Extra-
articular features are not common in early-stage RA.[3] As such, the presence
of certain extra-articular features may be used to rule out RA and diagnose
other conditions. For example, if there is skin, kidney, or lung involvement in
a patient with early-onset polyarthritis, one should look elsewhere for diagnostic possibilities including connective tissue diseases or the various forms
of systemic vasculitis.

*Rule 5: Symptoms out of proportion to physical findings facilitate differential diag-
nosis.* This rule applies primarily to connective tissue diseases and is rarely
applicable to RA.[3] For example, the patient with systemic lupus erythematosus will typically experience pain out of proportion to physical findings of
inflammation (warm, swollen, or tender joints). This rule also applies to the
fibromyalgia patient, since there are no findings of inflammation yet there is
widespread pain.

The implications of a diagnosis of RA have changed over the years. In today's
world, standard of care requires (see Chapter 11 on management) an aggressive approach for newly diagnosed RA patients, especially those with signs of a
poor prognosis, or for those who have had their signs and symptoms for a while
but have not sought medical help. Does this means that these patients should
be referred to a rheumatologist for management? The answer to this question
depends on the health care environment. In a perfect world, the answer should
be "yes." At a minimum, there should be a consultation and the development
of a communication strategy between the rheumatologist and the primary care
physician.

References

1. Arnett FC, Edworthy SM, Bloch DA, et al. The American Rheumatism Association 1987 revised criteria for the classification of rheumatoid arthritis. *Arthritis Rheum* 1988;31(3):315–324.

2. Kent PD, Matteson EL. Clinical features and differential diagnosis. In St. Clair EM, Pisetsky DS, Haynes BF, eds., *Rheumatoid Arthritis*. Philadelphia: Lippincott, Williams & Wilkins 2004;11–25.

3. van der Helm-van Mil, le Cessie S, Van Dongen H, et al. A prediction rule for disease outcome in patients with recent-onset undifferentiated arthritis: How to guide individual treatment decisions. *Arthritis Rheum* 2007;56(2):433–440.

4. Weisman MH, Corr MP. Differential diagnosis of acute and chronic polyarthritis. In Weisman MH, Weinblatt ME, Louie JS, eds., *Treatment of the rheumatic diseases: Companion to Kelley's textbook of rheumatology*, 2nd edition. Philadelphia: W.B. Saunders, 2001;4–29.

Chapter 11

Medications to Manage Rheumatoid Arthritis

The primary goals in treating patients with rheumatoid arthritis (RA) are to reduce pain and stiffness, slow disease progression (prevent damage), and improve function. For every individual patient, these three goals may have a different rank order of priority. Some patients can deal with whatever pain they have as long as they know that the progression of the disease is being treated; other patients will take the opposing view—stop the pain regardless of whether the drugs have a benefit regarding disease progression. Fortunately, the current availability of nonbiologic and biologic disease-modifying antirheumatic drugs (DMARDs) makes pain relief and the delay of disease progression a realistic possibility, while at the same time minimizing the toxicities associated with nonsteroidal anti-inflammatory drugs (NSAIDs) and corticosteroids.[1]

Treatment should be initiated as soon as a diagnosis of RA is made. Current recommendations suggest initiating treatment with methotrexate (the most well studied and effective nonbiologic DMARD) and an NSAID with or without corticosteroids to control symptoms.[1] Table 11.1 provides a list of treatment options, recommended usual dosage, and drug-specific adverse effects.

Nonsteroidal Anti-inflammatory Drugs

NSAIDs are used to control the pain experienced by patients with RA. In selecting an NSAID, the clinician should keep in mind the well-known risk for gastrointestinal adverse reactions and the fact that no particular NSAID is consistently more effective than any other.[1] Other side effects include renal toxicity, potential cardiovascular risk, and uncommonly, central nervous system effects.[1] Use of a flexible dosing regimen may reduce the occurrence of adverse events.[2] Patients not able to tolerate the gastrointestinal side effects of traditional NSAIDs may benefit from a cyclo-oxygenase (COX)-2 inhibitor. Although useful for controlling pain, there is no evidence that NSAIDs by themselves retard radiographic progression.[2] The overall use of NSAIDs in RA has declined in recent years, largely due to increased disease control with biologic agents and methotrexate. The concern over NSAID gastrointestinal toxicity and the oft-cited deaths attributed to the use of these agents have declined with improved disease control and less reliance on these agents in addition to increased awareness of safety concerns.

Corticosteroids

An estimated 25%–75% of patients with RA receive corticosteroid treatment[3] in spite of the fact that its use as a treatment strategy is controversial.[1] Systemically administered corticosteroids are an effective means of controlling painful synovitis, and intra-articular injections are extraordinarily useful for relieving acutely inflamed joints with minimal side effects.[1] There is some incontrovertible clinical trial evidence that 7.5 mg daily of prednisone retards radiographic progression.[1] Side effects associated with long-term use of corticosteroids include osteoporosis, weight gain, fluid retention, cataracts, glaucoma, poor wound healing, gastric ulcers and GI bleeding, hyperglycemia, hypertension, adrenal suppression, and increased risk of infection.[1] Every time a patient is placed on a corticosteroid, there should be a concomitant and simultaneously developed plan of action to taper and discontinue the drug in the future. In other words, you should not start this drug unless you have a plan of action to take the patient off of it.

The European League Against Rheumatism (EULAR) developed the following ten recommendations for the management of patients receiving corticosteroid treatment:[4]

1. The adverse effects of glucocorticoid therapy should be considered and discussed with the patient before glucocorticoid therapy is started.
2. Initial dose, dose reduction, and long-term dosing depend on the underlying rheumatic disease, disease activity, risk factors, and individual responsiveness of the patient.
3. When it is decided to start glucocorticoid treatment, comorbidities and risk factors for adverse effects should be evaluated and treated where indicated. These include hypertension, diabetes, peptic ulcer, recent fractures, presence of cataract or glaucoma, presence of (chronic) infections, dyslipidemia, and co-medication with NSAIDs.
4. For prolonged treatment, the glucocorticoid dosage should be kept to a minimum, and a glucocorticoid taper should be attempted in case of remission or low disease activity. The reasons to continue glucocorticoid therapy should be checked regularly.
5. During treatment, patients should be monitored for body weight, blood pressure, peripheral edema, cardiac insufficiency, serum lipids, blood and/or urine glucose, and ocular pressure depending on individual patient's risk, glucocorticoid dose and duration.
6. If a patient is started on prednisone >7.5 mg daily and continues on prednisone for more than 3 months, calcium and vitamin D supplementation should be prescribed. Antiresorptive therapy with bisphosphonates to reduce the risk of glucocorticoid-induced osteoporosis should be based on risk factors, including bone-mineral density (BMD) measurement.
7. Patients treated with glucocorticoids and concomitant NSAIDs should be given appropriate gastroprotective medication, such as proton pump inhibitors (PPIs) or misoprostol, or alternatively could switch to a COX-2 selective inhibitor (Coxib).

8. All patients on glucocorticoid therapy for longer than 1 month, who will undergo surgery, need perioperative management with adequate glucocorticoid replacement to overcome potential adrenal insufficiency.

9. Glucocorticoids during pregnancy have no additional risk for mother and child.

10. Children receiving glucocorticoids should be checked regularly for linear growth and considered for growth-hormone replacement in case of growth impairment.

Disease-modifying Antirheumatic Drugs

There are two classes of DMARDs: nonbiologics and biologics. Methotrexate and leflunomide are nonbiologics and are recommended by the American College of Rheumatology (ACR) as the first line of treatment for patients with RA of any duration and any degree of disease activity.[5] Methotrexate is typically well tolerated, but its side effects include stomatitis, anorexia, nausea, abdominal cramps, increased aminotransferase activity, and, in rare instances, hepatic fibrosis.[1] Leflunomide can be used as an alternative to methotrexate for patients who do not respond adequately or cannot tolerate the latter.[1] Adverse effects of leflunomide include diarrhea, reversible alopecia, rash, myelosuppression, and increases in aminotransferase activity. Hydroxychloroquine or sulfasalazine, either alone or in combination, are preferred by some clinicians for use in patients with mild RA.[1] The use of multiple DMARDs in combination may be indicated for use in patients with highly active disease, prolonged disease duration, and with clinical features portending a poor prognosis.[1] So-called "triple therapy" is a combination of methotrexate, sulfasalazine, and hydroxychloroquine—some investigators and clinicians prefer to use this combination before proceeding to a biologic agent. Whether or not the three-drug (or any nonbiologic) combination is superior to a biologic plus methotrexate is an open debate within the rheumatology community, but recent evidence indicates that the addition of a biologic agent to an incomplete methotrexate responder is superior (clinically and radiologically) to the addition of hydroxychloroquine plus sulfasalazine.[6]

The biologics, which are generally prescribed for patients with moderate to severe RA,[1] include tumor necrosis factor (TNF) inhibitors (golimumab, certolizumab pegol, etanercept, infliximab, adalimumab), a CD-20 monoclonal antibody (rituximab), a T-cell activation inhibitor (abatacept), an interleukin (IL)-1 receptor antagonist (anakinra), and an IL-6 receptor antagonist (tocilizumab). Of the biologics, anakinra is considered the least effective and is rarely used in clinical practice.[1] Treatment with TNF inhibitors, particularly when combined with methotrexate, significantly delays the progression of joint damage.[7] Patients receiving combination therapy demonstrate greater benefits than do patients receiving methotrexate monotherapy or TNF-blocker monotherapy.[7] In general, the ACR recommends using biologic DMARDs only after lack of adequate response to nonbiologic DMARDs.[5] However, the use of combination therapy with methotrexate and a TNF inhibitor should be considered for patients with early RA who exhibit high disease activity with a duration of any length (even <3 months), and a poor prognosis.[5]

Although injection site reactions are common with etanercept and adalimumab and infusion reactions may occur with infliximab, the most serious consequence of TNF inhibitors is the risk of severe infections and malignancies.[1] All analyses are confounded by the fact that both infections and malignancies occur in RA, regardless of treatment status. Randomized controlled trials in general during the drug approval process did not indicate a significant increased risk; however, meta-analyses, registry data, and other safety data reports published subsequent to the introduction of biologics show evidence of an increased incidence of severe and nonsevere infections, and some malignancies, although the findings are inconsistent.[8] For example, one meta-analysis of infliximab and adalimumab reported an increase risk for severe infections, whereas a meta-analysis of etanercept did not confirm an increased risk when used at recommended doses. Data from biologic registries, on the other hand, record the occurrence of both severe and nonsevere infections, as well as malignancies, among patients with RA treated with conventional DMARDs as well as TNF inhibitors.[8] It does appear from epidemiologic registry surveillance data that the increased risk of serious infections or malignancies occur very close to the time the biologic drug is administered.[9] These data suggest that the increased risk may relate to the presence of a subclinical disease that is "unmasked" by the biologic agent. One of the most common infections associated with the use of biologics is tuberculosis (TB), and the story here is the same as for other infections—latent TB appears to be unmasked by the biologic agent. As a result, it is recommended that patients be screened for TB (and treated for such) prior to initiating treatment with any biologic agent.[8] Because of the risk of infections during treatment with DMARDs, coupled with the fact that patients with RA are already immunocompromised, influenza and pneumococcal vaccinations are recommended prior to treatment.[1]

Treatment Strategies

State-of-the-art management of RA by rheumatologists in the 21st century has taken a welcome turn toward the early institution of aggressive management. In addition, rheumatologists have begun to recognize the importance of smoking cessation as an integral part of patient management. A variety of studies using real-world strategy designs[10–13] support the employment of treatment regimens that literally "knock-down" disease activity to a low level within weeks to months of initiation; if the low disease activity or clinical remission is not achieved immediately, patients receive an escalation of treatment strategies until this low disease activity is achieved. Most rheumatologists give methotrexate for 3 months to achieve its maximum effect and tolerability; if it is not achieved, patients then receive a biologic agent. This process will be accelerated if the patient has risk factors for a poor prognosis—a positive rheumatoid factor (RF) or antibody to cyclic citrullinated peptide (CCP). However, by this time, the RA patient is usually referred to a rheumatologist for advice and assistance in management.

Table 11.1 Current RA Treatments[1]

Class	Generic name	Usual Dose (generic)	Drug Specific Adverse Effects
Nonsteroidal Anti-Inflammatory Drugs			
Traditional NSAIDs	Diclofenac	150–200 mg/d in 2 or 3 doses	Increased thrombotic risk
	Extended release	100 mg once/d	
	Diflunisal	500–1000 mg/d in 2 does	
	Etodolac	300 mg bid–tid	
	Extended release	400 mg once/d	
	Fenoprofen	300–600 mg tid–qid	
	Flurbiprofen	200–300 mg/d in two, three, or four doses	
	Ibuprofen	1600–3200 mg/d in three or four doses	Slight increased thrombotic risk
	Indomethacin	50 mg tid–qid	Increased thrombotic risk
	Extended release	75 mg once/d or bid	
	Ketoprofen	50 mg quid or 75 mg tid	
	Extended release	200 mg once/d	
	Meclofenamate sodium	200–400 mg/d in three or four doses	
	Meloxicam	7.5–15 mg once/d	Increased thrombotic risk
	Nabumetone	1,000–2,000 mg/d in one or two doses	
	Naproxen	250–500 mg bid–tid	
	Naproxen sodium	275 mg or 550 mg bid	
	Oxaprozin	1,200 mg once/d	
	Piroxicam	20 mg once/d	Slight increased thrombotic risk

continued

Table 11.1 Continued

Class	Generic name	Usual Dose (generic)	Drug Specific Adverse Effects
	Sulindac	150–200 mg bid	
	Tolmetin	600–1,800 mg/d in three or four doses	
COX-2 inhibitor	Celecoxib	100–200 mg bid	Less upper GI toxicity than nonselective NSAIDs
Salicylates, acetylated	Aspirin, extended-release	800 mg qid	
	Aspirin, enteric-coated	975 mg qid	
Salicylates, non-acetylated	Choline magnesium trisalicylate	3 g/d in one, two, or three doses	
	Salicylsalicylic acid (salsalate)	3–4 g/d in two or three doses	
Glucocorticoids			
	Prednisone	5–7.5 mg daily	
	Triamcinolone	Intra-articular injection	
	Methylprednisolone	Intra-articular injection	
Disease-modifying Antirheumatic Drugs			
Nonbiologics	Methotrexate, oral	7.5–25 mg once/wk PO	Stomatitis, anorexia, nausea, abdominal cramps, increased aminotransferase activity and, rarely, hepatic fibrosis
	Methotrexate, injectable	7.5–25 mg once/wk IM or SC	
	Hydroxychloroquine sulfate	200–400 mg/d PO	Nausea and epigastric pain; possible immediate blurred vision or difficulty seeing at night
	Sulfasalazine	2–3 g/d in divided doses PO	Nausea, anorexia, and rash
	Leflunomide	10–20 mg/d PO	Diarrhea, reversible alopecia, rash, myelosuppression, and increases in aminotransferase activity
	Gold salts	50 mg/wk IM	Stomatitis, rash, proteinuria and less commonly, leukopenia and thrombocytopenia

	Dose	Adverse Effects
Azathioprine	1–2.5 mg/kg once/d or in divided doses PO	GI intolerance, hepatitis, bone marrow suppression; reports of increased risk of lymphoma
Cyclosporine	2.5–4 mg/kg/d PO	Nephrotoxicity and interactions with drugs and foods
Minocycline	50–200 mg/d in divided doses PO	Drug-induced lupus
Biologics TNF Inhibitors Etanercept	25 mg 2x/wk or 50 mg once/wk SC	Injection site reactions
Infliximab	3 mg/kg at 0, 2, and 6 wks, then every 8 wks IV	Infusion reactions including fever, urticaria, dyspnea, and hypotension
Adalimumab	40 mg q1–2 wks SC	Injection site reactions
Golimumab	50 mg SC once monthly	FDA black box warning regarding the potential for reactivation of tuberculosis and invasive fungal infections
Certolizumab pegol	400 mg (given as two subcutaneous injections of 200 mg) at weeks 0, 2, and 4, followed by a maintenance dose of 200 mg every 2 weeks or 400 mg every 4 weeks	FDA black box warning regarding the potential for reactivation of tuberculosis and invasive fungal infections
CD monoclonal antibody Rituximab	1,000 mg IV twice, 2 weeks apart	Anaphylaxis and anaphylactoid reactions, progressive multifocal leukoencephalopathy due to JC virus infection, reactivation of hepatitis B infection
T-Cell activation inhibitor Abatacept	500, 750, or 1,000 mg at 0, 2, and 4 weeks, then q4 weeks IV	Hypertension, headache, dizziness, and, rarely, anaphylactoid reactions
IL-1 receptor antagonist Anakinra	100 mg/d SC	Injection site reactions
IL-6 receptor antagonist Tocilizumab	4 mg/kg IV drip infusion every 4 weeks, followed by increase to 8 mg/kg based on clinical response	FDA black box warning regarding the potential for reactivation of tuberculosis and invasive fungal infections Upper respiratory tract infections, nasopharyngitis, headache, hypertension, and increased ALT have also been reported

Adapted from Drugs for Rheumatoid Arthritis. Treatment Guidelines from the Medical Letter 2009;7:37–46.

References

1. Drugs for rheumatoid arthritis. *Treatment Guidelines from the Medical Letter* 2009;7(81):37–46

2. Kvien TK. Nonsteroidal anti-inflammatory drugs and coxibs. In Hochberg MC et al., eds. *Rheumatoid Arthritis,* 1st edition. Philadelphia: Mosby 2009:295–299.

3. Bijlsma JW, Buttgereit F. Glucocorticoids. In Hochberg MC et al., eds. *Rheumatoid Arthritis,* 1st edition. Philadelphia: Mosby 2009:300–306.

4. Hoes JN, Jacobs JW, Boers M, et al. EULAR evidence-based recommendations on the management of systemic glucocorticoid therapy in rheumatic diseases. *Ann Rheum Dis* 2007;66(12):1560–1567.

5. Saag KG, Teng GG, Patkar NM, et al. American College of Rheumatology 2008 recommendations for the use of nonbiologic and biologic disease-modifying anti-rheumatic drugs in rheumatoid arthritis. *Arthritis Rheum* 2008;59(6):762–784.

6. van Vollenhoven RF, Ernestam S, Geborek P et al. Addition of infliximab compared with addition of sulfasalazine and hydroxychloroquine to methotrexate in patients with early rheumatoid arthritis (Swefot trial): 1-year results of a randomised trial. *Lancet* 2009;374(9688):459–466.

7. Smolen JS, Aletaha D, Koeller M, et al. New therapies for treatment of rheumatoid arthritis. *Lancet* 2007;370(9602):1861–1874.

8. Martin-Mola E, Balsa A. Infectious complications of biologic agents. *Rheum Dis Clin N Am* 2009;35(1):183–199.

9. Askling J, Baecklund E, Granath F, et al. Anti-tumour necrosis factor therapy in rheumatoid arthritis and risk of malignant lymphomas: Relative risks and time trends in the Swedish Biologics Register *Ann Rheum Dis* 2009;68(5):648–653.

10. Bakker MF, Jacobs JW, Verstappen SM, Bijlsma JW. Tight control in the treatment of rheumatoid arthritis: Efficacy and feasibility. *Ann Rheum Dis* 2007;66(Suppl 3):iii56–60.

11. Goekoop-Ruiterman YP, de Vries-Bouwstra JK, Allaart CF, et al. Clinical and radiographic outcomes of four different treatment strategies in patients with early rheumatoid arthritis (the BeSt study): A randomized, controlled trial. *Arthritis Rheum* 2005;52(11):3381–90.

12. Grigor C, Capell H, Stirling A, et al. Effect of a treatment strategy of tight control for rheumatoid arthritis (the TICORA study): A single-blind randomised controlled trial. *Lancet* 2004;364(9430):263–269.

13. Verstappen SM, Jacobs JW, van der Veen MJ, et al. Intensive treatment with methotrexate in early rheumatoid arthritis: Aiming for remission. Computer Assisted Management in Early Rheumatoid Arthritis (CAMERA, an open-label strategy trial). *Ann Rheum Dis* 2007;66(11):1443–1449.

Chapter 12

Economic Impact and Disability Issues

There are significant direct costs attendant with the treatment of rheumatoid arthritis (RA), as well as considerable indirect costs associated with the functional disability incurred by patients with RA. Direct costs include the cost of drugs, hospitalization, and outpatient procedures.[1] Indirect costs encompass productivity losses due to one's inability to work or engage in usual activities.[2] Estimates of direct and indirect costs should be viewed with caution, because of the variations in methodological procedures used to collect and analyze the data.[3]

The drug component of direct medical costs has increased substantially since the introduction of biologic disease-modifying antirheumatic drugs (DMARDs), the cost of which ranges between $10,000 and $20,000 annually,[4] more than triple the cost of traditional RA treatments.[5] Theoretically, the increase in the drug component of direct costs should be offset by a decrease in hospitalization and outpatient procedures, due to the ability of biologics to significantly retard disease progression. However, methodological issues render it difficult to estimate any potential cost savings due to early intervention with biologics.[6]

In a study undertaken subsequent to the introduction of biologic DMARDs, Michaud et al. reported on the direct costs of 7,527 patients in the United States who completed detailed self-report questionnaires as part of their participation in the National Data Bank for Rheumatic Diseases (NDB). In 2001, the mean annual direct cost for a patient with RA was $9,519: $6,324 (66%) for drug costs, $1,573 (17%) for hospitalization costs, and $1,541 (17%) for outpatient costs.[1] The mean annual direct cost for patients receiving biologic agents compared to patients not receiving biological agents was $19,016 and $6,164, respectively.[1] In contrast, Cooper completed a systematic review of the literature that included studies primarily from the United States, but also from Canada, the United Kingdom, the Netherlands, and Sweden prior to the widespread use of biologic DMARDs. The average annual direct medical cost ranged from $5,720 to $5,822, with drug costs comprising 8%–24% of the total, hospitalization between 17% and 88% of the total, and physician visits between 8% and 21% of the total.[3]

The course of RA is variable, and patients may experience limited to severe disease activity during various periods of their lives. Among patients with functional impairment, the consequences can be devastating, especially with regard to ability to function on the job. For example, among two cohorts of women newly diagnosed with RA, 31% of women diagnosed in 1987 stopped working during the 3-year follow-up period, whereas 26% of women diagnosed in 1998 stopped working during the follow-up period. Married women and women with joint deformities were more likely to stop working.[7]

Absenteeism and job cessation are significant factors contributing to the indirect cost of RA. One estimate places the average number of days absent from work at between 2.7 and 30 days per year.[3] The time from disease onset to work cessation is variable as well. Using data from the NDB, Allaire et al. calculated that the prevalence of arthritis-attributed work cessation increases with disease duration. Approximately 14% of patients with RA ceased work within 1–3 years of disease onset, 28.9% within 10 years of disease onset, and 42.2% after disease duration of 25 years or more.[8] A survival analysis derived from data included in a systematic review of the literature from several countries indicates that the time from disease onset until a 50% probability of work disability varies from 4.5 to 22 years, with a median of 13 years.[9] A review of the literature places estimates of the indirect cost of RA at a low of $760 in Thailand and a high of $32,155 in the United States.[2] Among studies conducted in the United States, indirect costs ranged from a low of $2,317 to a high of $32,155.[2] Given all of this information that has been collected as to the high societal cost of having RA, it is difficult to find accurate information about treatment strategies that may impact this cost. Data gleaned from clinical trials (many of these have been published) cannot accurately provide us with this information, since treatments are standardized in these studies and patient selection will affect the results. We await large-scale real-world effectiveness studies.

References

1. Michaud K, Messer J, Choi HK et al. Direct medical costs and their predictors in patients with rheumatoid arthritis: A three-year study of 7,527 patients. *Arthritis Rheum* 2003;48(10):2750–2762.

2. Xie F. The need for standardization: A literature review of indirect costs of rheumatoid arthritis and osteoarthritis. *Arthritis Rheum* 2008;59(7):1027–1033.

3. Cooper NJ. Economic burden of rheumatoid arthritis: A systematic review. *Rheumatology* 2000;39(1):28–33.

4. Solomon DH, Kavanaugh A. Pharmacoeconomic aspects of rheumatoid arthritis management. In Hochberg MC, et al., eds., *Rheumatoid Arthritis*, 1st edition. Philadelphia: Mosby 2009;285–288.

5. Tan MC, Regier DA, Esdaile JM, et al. Health economic evaluation: A primer for the practicing rheumatologist. *Arthritis Rheum* 2006;55(4):648–656.

6. Bansback N, Marra CA, Finckh A, Anis A. The economics of treatment in early rheumatoid arthritis. *Best Pract Res Clin Rheumatol* 2009;23(1):83–92.

7. Reisine S, Fifield J, Walsh S, Dauser D. Work disability among two cohorts of women with recent-onset rheumatoid arthritis: a survival analysis. *Arthritis Rheum* 2007;57(3):372–380.

8. Allaire S, Wolfe F, Niu J, LaValley MP. Contemporary prevalence and incidence of work disability associated with rheumatoid arthritis in the US. *Arthritis Rheum* 2008;59(4):474–480.

9. Burton W, Morrison A, Maclean R, Ruderman E. Systematic review of studies of productivity loss due to rheumatoid arthritis. *Occup Med* 2006;56(1):18–27.

Chapter 13

Prognosis

Our knowledge of the pathogenesis, natural history, and treatment of rheumatoid arthritis (RA) has significantly advanced over the last century since Sir Archibald Barring first designated RA as a distinct rheumatological entity in 1907.[1] Hench's discovery of cortisone provided hope that patients with RA could ultimately achieve remission.[2] Although that hope was dashed within a short period, the introduction of no fewer than nine targeted biologic agents within the last few years[3] continues to yield favorable results. Although by no means is the disease cured, when RA is detected early and the patient is treated immediately with disease-modifying antirheumatic drugs (DMARDs), the prognosis is quite promising. For RA patients in this time of methotrexate and biological therapy, a significantly improved outlook lies ahead. First, there is evidence of arrested disease progression[3] as well as disease remission in a small number of patients.[3,4] Second, biological agents have had a significant impact on quality of life and productivity.[5] Third, due to improved pharmacologic management of RA, the number of RA-related hospital admissions[6] and RA-related orthopedic and joint surgeries,[7,8] markers of disease severity, have decreased over the last 20 years. Finally, rehabilitation programs such as progressive resistance training[9] and occupational therapy,[10] heretofore unthinkable, have been tested as possible methods for delaying the onset of work disability. Probably the most important factor that has contributed to improved outcomes for RA patients is the recognition (and subsequent diminution) of the adverse effect of cigarette smoking on disease susceptibility and severity. The relationship between cigarette smoking, pathogenesis of RA, and genetic susceptibility for the disease is an ongoing research focus.[11]

The DMARDs, whether nonbiologic or biologic, are by no means a miracle cure for RA. However, they have been demonstrated to arrest disease progression and subsequent joint damage and, in a small number of cases, complete drug remission has been achieved. Remission rates vary with type of therapy, when it is instituted, and disease duration in the patient. In general, remission rates in patients treated with traditional, nonbiologic DMARD monotherapy range from 7% to 22% ,[12] whereas remission rates in patients treated with biologic combination therapy range from 13% to 42%.[12] Data from the STURE registry in Sweden indicate that in one study, 40% of patients with established RA achieved low disease activity, whereas only 24% achieved remission.[3] Four-year follow-up data from the Dutch BeSt study, a head-to-head comparison of four different treatment strategies implemented in patients with disease duration of less than 2 years, has just been published.[4] Drug-free remission was attained by 13% of patients, whereas remission measured by a DAS score of less than 1.6 was attained by 43%.[4] Variables identified by multivariate regression as being independently associated with drug-free remission were absence of anticyclic citrullinated peptide antibodies, male gender, and short symptom duration. Interestingly, treatment strategy was not independently associated with drug-free remission in the BeSt study.[4] The most likely explanation for the observed outcomes of these strategy approaches (as exemplified by the BeSt study) is not necessarily the drugs themselves but the timing of their implementation.

Ultimately, remission for the majority of patients with RA remains an elusive goal, and several important avenues of research require continued exploration. In time, it is possible that the further specification of pathogenic mechanisms, the identification of targeted therapeutics, and continued research into predictive biomarkers will yield new strategies for significantly controlling the debilitating effects of the disease and improving the quality of life of patients with RA.

Quality of Life and Productivity

A recent review by Strand and Singh[5] highlights improvements in health-related quality of life (HRQOL) and productivity attributed to biological treatments. Among the TNF inhibitors, for example, treatment with infliximab plus methotrexate for 2 years resulted in significant improvements in both the physical and mental health component of the SF-36 score, a generic quality-of-life measure, for patients enrolled in the ATTRACT trial.[5] In the AIM trial, patients receiving abatacept, a costimulatory molecule inhibitor, plus methotrexate reported statistically significant improvements in each of the eight SF-36 domains compared to patients receiving placebo plus methotrexate.[5] In the same review, Strand and Singh report similar improvements in productivity related to treatment with biological agents. In the ASPIRE trial, employed patients receiving combination therapy reported significantly fewer lost workdays compared to patients receiving monotherapy.[5] Furthermore, at 1 year, 8% of patients treated with infliximab plus methotrexate became unemployed, compared to 14% receiving monotherapy.[5] These examples and data from other clinical trials provide unequivocal evidence that treatment of RA with biological agents is associated with improvements in HRQOL and productivity.

RA-related Hospital Admissions and RA-related Orthopedic and Joint Surgeries

As a consequence of severe disease, RA patients may find themselves hospitalized and/or facing orthopedic procedures or joint replacement surgery. A growing body of evidence suggests that hospitalizations and surgeries for patients with RA have decreased or shown no significant increase since the introduction of DMARD therapy. The design of these studies do not allow us to conclude with certainty that DMARD therapy is directly responsible for the decline in hospitalizations and surgeries, but the results are strong enough to not dismiss the possibility that this may be the case.

Ward[6] studied changes in the rates of hospitalization for four manifestations of severe RA: rheumatoid vasculitis, splenectomy for Felty's syndrome, cervical spine fusion for myelopathy, and total knee arthroplasty. Using data from the California hospital discharge database for 1983–2001, he found that the risk for hospitalization for rheumatoid vasculitis had decreased by one-third for the period 1998–2001 compared to 1983–1987. The risk of hospitalization for splenectomy in Felty's syndrome was 71% lower over the same time intervals. Although rates of hospitalization for cervical spine surgery or total knee arthroplasty did not decrease, there was a reversal of the trend of increasing rates of total knee arthroplasty.[6] Several studies from around the world document the decline in the number of orthopedic and joint surgeries among patients with RA. For example, in the United States, a retrospective medical review of RA incident cases in Rochester, Minnesota, during 1955–1995 found that patients diagnosed with RA after 1985 were significantly less likely to have undergone joint surgery for RA than those diagnosed prior to 1985.[7] Weiss et al.[8] report that in Sweden, lower limb orthopedic surgery showed a consistent decrease over the period 1987–2001. At the same time, rates of RA-related upper limb surgery significantly decreased over the period 1998–2004. Although not definitive, these studies suggest that patients newly diagnosed with arthritis face a somewhat altered landscape from their earlier predecessors, with a reduced rate of complications from their RA.

Rehabilitation Programs

Recently, novel approaches to the treatment of RA-related physical deficits have been attempted in an effort to improve muscle mass and functional outcomes. Lemmey et al.[9] conducted a small ($N = 28$) randomized controlled trial to test the effectiveness of high-intensity progressive resistance training compared to range-of-movement home exercises in restoring muscle mass and function in patients with RA. At the conclusion of the 24-week trial, patients who participated in progressive resistance training significantly increased their lean body mass and physical function compared to patients participating in the home exercise condition. Although seemingly suggesting that RA patients should begin resistance training exercises, it is important to note that the patients participating in this study had low disease activity levels. Furthermore, it remains to be determined whether progressive resistance training is possible in patients with more advanced disease.

A trial aimed at improving functional outcomes and averting work disability among employed RA patients compared a 6-month occupational therapy regimen with usual care.[10] Several functional outcome measures were included in the evaluation including, among others, the Canadian Occupational Performance Measure (COPM), the Health Assessment Questionnaire (HAQ), and the RA Work Instability Scale (WIS). Multivariate analysis confirmed improvements in physical function for patients in the occupational therapy group for the COPM and the HAQ, but not for the RA WIS.[10] Although certainly subject to interpretation, the outlook for the RA patient facing the possibility of work-related disability has been significantly changed for the better.

References

1. Symmons DP. What is rheumatoid arthritis? *Br. Med Bull* 1995;51(2):243–248.

2. Glyn J. The discovery and early use of cortisone. *J R Soc Med* 1998; 91(10):513–517.

3. van Vollenhoven RF. Treatment of rheumatoid arthritis: state of the art 2009. *Nat Rev Rheumatol* 2009;5(10):531–541.

4. van der Kooij SM, Goekoop-Ruiterman YP, de Vries-Bouwstra JK, et al. Drug free remission, functioning and radiographic damage after 4 years of response-driven treatment in patients with recent-onset rheumatoid arthritis. *Ann Rheum Dis* 2009;68(6):914–921.

5. Strand V, Singh J. Newer biological agents in rheumatoid arthritis: Impact on health-related quality of life and productivity. *Drugs* 2010;70(2):121–145.

6. Ward MM. Decreases in rates of hospitalizations for manifestations of severe rheumatoid arthritis, 1983–2001. *Arthritis Rheum* 2004;50(4):1122–1131.

7. da Silva E, Doran MF, Crowson CS, et al. Declining use of orthopedic surgery in patients with rheumatoid arthritis? Results of a long-term, population-based assessment. *Arthritis Rheum* 2003;49(2):216–220.

8. Weiss RJ, Ehlin A, Montgomery SM, et al. Decrease of RA-related orthopaedic surgery of the upper limbs between 1998 and 2004: Data from 54579 Swedish RA inpatients. *Rheumatology* 2008;47(4):491–494.

9. Lemmey AB, Marcora SM, Chester K, et al. Effects of high-intensity resistance training in patients with rheumatoid arthritis: A randomized controlled trial. *Arthritis Rheum* 2009;61(12):1726–1734.

10. Macedo AM, Oakley SP, Panayi GS, Kirkham BW. Functional and work outcomes improve in patients with rheumatoid arthritis who receive targeted, comprehensive occupational therapy. *Arthritis Rheum* 2009;61(11):1522–1530.

11. Baka Z, Buzás E, Nagy G. Rheumatoid arthritis and smoking: Putting the pieces together. *Arthritis Res Ther* 2009;11(4):238.

12. Sesin CA, Bingham CO. Remission in rheumatoid arthritis: Wishful thinking or clinical reality? *Semin Arthritis Rheum* 2005;35(3):185–196.

Glossary

ACR The America College of Rheumatology, formerly known as the ARA (American Rheumatism Association). A professional association of 4,000 American rheumatologists, of whom 2,800 are board certified. Criteria, or definitions, for many rheumatic diseases are referred to as ACR criteria.

AIMS Arthritis Impact Measurement Scales.

ACPA Anti-citrullinated protein antibodies frequently detected in patients with RA.

Allele One member of a pair or series of different forms of a gene. An allele is usually a coding sequence.

Antibodies Special protein substances made by the body's white blood cells for defense against bacteria and other foreign substances.

Anti-inflammatory Agent that counteracts or suppresses inflammation.

Antigen A substance that prompts the generation of antibodies and can cause an immune response.

APC Antigen-presenting cells, such as B cells, dendritic cells, or macrophages, that lead to the activation of autoreactive T lymphocytes.

Articular surface The surface of a joint at which the ends of the bones meet.

Autoantibody Antibody to one's own tissues or cells.

B cell A lymphocyte involved in immune regulation.

BAL Bronchoalveolar lavage.

Biologics Targeted immune therapies.

BMI Body mass index. Defined as an individual's body weight divided by the square of his or her height.

CCP Cyclic citrullinated peptide. A peptide that incorporates the amino acid citrulline.

CDAI Clinical Disease Activity Index.

CLINHAQ Clinical Health Assessment Questionnaire.

Corticosteroid Any natural anti-inflammatory hormone made by the adrenal cortex; may also be made synthetically.

CP-690,550 A small molecule JAK antagonist currently being tested in clinical trials for the treatment of RA.

CRP C-reactive protein. An acute-phase protein found in the blood, the levels of which rise in response to inflammation.

CT Computed tomography.

CVD Cardiovascular disease.

Cytokines Group of signaling molecules that are used extensively in cellular communication.

DAS Disease Activity Scores. The DAS is a measure of the activity of rheumatoid arthritis and includes a count of tender and swollen joints, and may include measures of CRP or ESR.

DMARD Disease-modifying antirheumatic drug, the purpose of which is to inhibit disease progression.

ESR Erythrocyte sedimentation rate. A nonspecific measure of inflammation.

EULAR European League Against Rheumatism. A professional organization that aims to promote, stimulate, and support the research, prevention, treatment, and rehabilitation of rheumatic diseases.

ExRA Extra-articular manifestations of RA.

HAQ Health Assessment Questionnaire. An outcome measure designed to measure functional status and disability in patients with rheumatoid arthritis and other rheumatological diseases.

HLA Histocompatibility locus antigen. Molecules inside a macrophage that bind to an antigenic peptide. Controlled by genes on the sixth chromosome. They can amplify or perpetuate certain immune and inflammatory responses.

HLA-DR Histocompatibility locus antigen direct repeat.

HRQOL Health-related quality of life.

IDDM Insulin-dependent diabetes mellitus

IHD Ischemic heart disease.

IIP Idiopathic interstitial pneumonia.

ILD Interstitial lung disease.

IMT Carotid artery intima–media thickness.

Inflammation Swelling, heat, and redness resulting from the infiltration of white blood cells into tissues.

IP Interstitial pneumonitis.

JAK/STAT Janus Kinase/Signal Transducer and Activator of Transcription. JAKs are members of a family of cytoplasmic protein tyrosine kinases that have a significant influence in mediating inflammatory immune responses.

Lymphocyte Type of white blood cell that fights infection and mediates the immune response.

Macrophage White blood cells that kill foreign material and present information to lymphocytes.

MACTAR McMaster Toronto Arthritis Patient Preference Disability Questionnaire.

MCP Metacarpophalangeal joint. Located in fingers and thumbs.

MCP-1 Monocyte chemotactic protein.

MCSF Macrophage colony-stimulating factor.

MDHAQ Multidimensional Health Assessment Questionnaire.

MHC Major histocompatibility complex. Same as HLA.

MMP Matrix metalloproteinases. A member of a group of enzymes that are able to break down proteins that are normally found in the spaces between cells in tissues.

MRI Magnetic resonance imaging.

MTP Metatarsophalangeal joint. Joints between the metatarsal bones of the foot and the proximal bones of the toes.

NHANES III Third National Health and Nutrition Examination Survey. A survey conducted under the auspices of the National Center for Health Statistics designed to measure the health and nutritional status of adults and children in the United States.

NSAID Nonsteroidal anti-inflammatory drug that fights inflammation by blocking the actions of prostaglandin.

NSIP Nonspecific interstitial pneumonia.

OA Osteoarthritis.

OCP Oral contraceptive pill.

PIP Proximal interphalangeal joint. Hinge joints of the phalanges of the hand.

R406 An inhibitor of SyK kinase.

R788 The prodrug of R406 that is being test as a potential new therapeutic target for the treatment of RA.

RANKL Receptor activator for nuclear factor κ B-ligand.

RAQOL Rheumatoid Arthritis Quality of Life. A disease-specific quality-of-life measure.

RF Rheumatoid factor. An immunoglobulin (antibody) that can bind to other antibodies.

SDAI Simplified Disease Activity Index.

SE Shared epitope. A common stretch of amino acids in the peptide-binding grooves at positions 67–74 of the HLA-DR β-chain.

SENS Simple erosion narrowing score.

SF-36 Short Form 36. A generic measure of health-related quality of life.

SLE Systemic lupus erythematosus. A chronic, inflammatory autoimmune disorder that may affect the skin, joints, kidneys, and other organs.

SyK Spleen tyrosine kinase, an important regulator of cell signaling.

Synovial fluid Joint fluid.

Synovitis Inflammation of the tissues lining a joint.

Synovium Tissue that lines a joint.

T1D Type 1 diabetes. An autoimmune disease that results in destruction of insulin-producing beta cells of the pancreas.

T Cell Lymphocyte responsible for immunologic memory.

TMJ Temporomandibular joint, a jaw joint.

TNF Tumor necrosis factor, formally known as tumor necrosis factor-α, is a cytokine involved in systemic inflammation and is a member of a group of cytokines that stimulate the acute phase reaction.

UIP Usual interstitial pneumonia.

US Ultrasound.

Rheumatoid Arthritis Resource Materials

What organizations provide patient support in the United States?

Although many organizations provide patient support for rheumatoid arthritis (RA) in the United States, only those with a budget of over $1 million are listed.

American Autoimmune Related Diseases Associations (AARDA)
National Office
22100 Gratiot Avenue
East Detroit, MI 48021
Phone: 586-776-3900
Web site: www.aarda.org

Arthritis Foundation
PO Box 7669
Atlanta, GA 30357
Phone: 800-283-7800
Web site: www.arthritis.org

Each state in the United States has at least one, if not multiple chapters, that provide research funding, publish literature, and offer patient support for rheumatoid arthritis.

Where can I find reliable information about RA?

American College of Rheumatology (ACR)
1800 Century Place
Suite 250
Atlanta, GA 30345
Phone: 404–633-3777
Web site: www.rheumatology.org

This is the professional organization to which nearly all U.S. and many international rheumatologists belong.

National Institute of Arthritis and Musculoskeletal and Skin Diseases (NIAMS)
Building 31, Room 4C02
31 Center Drive - MSC 2350
Bethesda, MD 20892
Phone: 301-496-8190
Web site: www.niams.nih.gov

Part of the National Institutes of Health, NIAMS allocated approximately $135 million to rheumatoid arthritis research in 2009.

What other organizations fund RA research?

Arthritis National Research Foundation
200 Oceangate, Suite 830
Long Beach, CA 90802
Phone: 800-588-2873
Web site: www.curearthritis.org

How can I find out about arthritis support outside of the United States?

The Arthritis Society, Canada
National Office
393 University Avenue, Suite 1700
Toronto, Ontario M5G 1E6
Canada
Phone: 416-979-7228
Web site: www.arthritis.ca

Arthritis Care, United Kingdom
18 Stephenson Way
London NW1 2HD
Phone: 020-7380-6500
Web site: www.arthritiscare.org.uk

Rheumatoid Arthritis Text books

Hochberg MC, Silman AJ, Smolen JS, Weinblatt ME, Weisman MH, eds. *Rheumatoid Arthritis,* 1st edition, Philadelphia: Mosby, 2009.

General Rheumatology Textbooks

Weisman MH, Weinblatt ME, Louie JS, Van Vollenhoven RF. *Targeted treatment of the rheumatic diseases.* Philadelphia: W.B. Saunders, 2010.

Hochberg MC, Silman AJ, Smolen JS, Weinblatt ME, Weisman MH. *Rheumatology.* 4th edition. Philadelphia: Mosby 2008.

HAQ-DI Disability Index

The STANFORD HEALTH ASSESSMENT QUESTIONNAIRE©
Stanford University School of Medicine
Division of Immunology & Rheumatology

<u>HAQ Disability Index</u>

In this section we are interested in learning how your illness affects your ability to function in daily life. Please feel free to add any comments on the back of this page.

Please check the response which best describes your usual abilities OVER THE PAST WEEK:

	Without ANY difficulty[0]	With SOME difficulty[1]	With MUCH difficulty[2]	UNABLE to do[3]
Dressing & Grooming				
Are you able to:				
-Dress yourself, including tying shoelaces and doing buttons?	☐	☐	☐	☐
-Shampoo your hair?	☐	☐	☐	☐
ARISING				
Are you able to:				
-Stand up from a straight chair?	☐	☐	☐	☐
-Get in and out of bed?	☐	☐	☐	☐
EATING				
Are you able to:				
-Cut your meat?	☐	☐	☐	☐
-Lift a full cup or glass to your mouth	☐	☐	☐	☐
-Open a new milk carton?	☐	☐	☐	☐
WALKING				
Are you able to:				
-Walk outdoors on flat ground?	☐	☐	☐	☐
-Climb up five steps?	☐	☐	☐	☐

Please check any AIDS OR DEVICES that you usually use for any of these activities:

☐ Cane
☐ Walker
☐ Crutches
☐ Wheelchair

☐ Devices used for dressing (button hook, zipper pul long-handled shoe horn, etc.)
☐ Built up or special utensils
☐ Special or built up chair
☐ Other (Specify:_____)

Please check any categories for which you usually need HELP FROM ANOTHER PERSON:

☐ Dressing and Grooming
☐ Arising

☐ Eating
☐ Walking

Please check the response which best describes your usual abilities **OVER THE PAST WEEK:**

	Without ANY difficulty[0]	With SOME difficulty[1]	With MUCH difficulty[2]	UNABLE to do[3]
HYGIENE				
Are you able to:				
-Wash and dry your body?	☐	☐	☐	☐
-Take a tub bath?	☐	☐	☐	☐
-Get on and off the toilet?	☐	☐	☐	☐
REACH				
Are you able to:				
-Reach and get down a 5-pound object (such as a bag of sugar) from just above your head?	☐	☐	☐	☐
-Bend down to pick up clothing from the floor?	☐	☐	☐	☐
GRIP				
Are you able to:				
-Open car doors?	☐	☐	☐	☐
-Open jars which have been previously opened?	☐	☐	☐	☐
-Turn faucets on and off?	☐	☐	☐	☐
ACTIVITIES				
Are you able to:				
-Run errands and shop?	☐	☐	☐	☐
-Get in and out of a car?	☐	☐	☐	☐
-Do chores such as vacuuming or yardwork	☐	☐	☐	☐

Please check any AIDS OR DEVICES that you usually use for any of these activities:

☐ Raised toilet seat
☐ Bathtub seat
☐ Jar opener (for jars previously opened)

☐ Bathtub bar
☐ Long-handled appliances for reach
☐ Long-handled appliances in bathroom
☐ Other (Specify: _____)

Please check any categories for which you usually need HELP FROM ANOTHER PERSON:

☐ Hygiene
☐ Reach

☐ Gripping and opening things
☐ Errands and chores

We are also interested in learning whether or not you are affected by pain because of your illness. **How much pain have you had because of your illness IN THE PAST WEEK:**

PLACE A <u>VERTICAL</u> (|) MARK ON THE LINE TO INDICATE THE SEVERITY OF THE PAIN

No Pain   **Severe Pain**

0   100

Considering all the ways that your arthritis affects you, rate how you are doing on the following scale by placing a vertical mark on the line.

Very Well   **Very Poor**

0   100

Index

87